Ethics and Aging

This book is an important and timely look at issues of ethics in aging. It reflects the complexity of these questions, but develops them in relation to a single general theme: that of the involvement of the elderly in the design of social policy and the research which affects them.

Moral problems involving the elderly are many-faceted. Accurate understanding and social response demand some integration of experience, sensibility, and knowledge provided by different perspectives. *Ethics and Aging* incorporates viewpoints from gerontology, philosophy, law, theology, sociology, psychology, medicine, nursing, and economics.

JAMES E. THORNTON is coordinator, Committee on Gerontology, the University of British Columbia.

EARL R. WINKLER is an associate professor in the department of philosophy at the University of British Columbia.

Ethics and Aging:
THE RIGHT TO LIVE, THE RIGHT TO DIE

Edited by James E. Thornton
and Earl R. Winkler
Assisted by Megan Stuart-Stubbs

THE UNIVERSITY OF BRITISH COLUMBIA PRESS
VANCOUVER 1988

Printed in Canada

ISBN (cloth) 0-7748-0302-9
ISBN (paper) 0-7748-0310-X

Canadian Cataloguing in Publication Data

Main entry under title:

Ethics and aging

Bibliography: p.
Includes index.

ISBN 0-7748-0302-9 (bound). — ISBN 0–7748–0310–X (pbk.)

1. Aging – Moral and ethical aspects. 2. Aged – Social conditions. I. Thornton, James E. (James Edward), 1927- II. Winkler, Earl R. (Earl Raye), 1938-
HQ1061.E83 1988 305.2′6 C88-091471-8

This book has been published with the help of a grant from the Canadian Federation for the Humanities, using funds provided by the Social Sciences and Humanities Research Council of Canada.

Contents

Acknowledgments / vii
Contributors / ix

1 Introduction to Principal Themes and Issues / 3
EARL R. WINKLER AND JAMES E. THORNTON

PART ONE: GENERAL PERSPECTIVES

2 On Reaching a New Agenda: Self-Determination and Aging / 16
JANE A. BOYAJIAN

3 Ethics and Aging: Trends and Problems in the Clinical Setting / 31
DAVID ROY

4 Ethical Aspects of Aging: Justice, Freedom, and Responsibility / 41
JOHN C. BENNETT

5 Paradigms of Aging: Growth versus Decline / 54
JAMES E. BIRREN AND CANDACE A. STACEY

6 Cognitive Intervention in Later Life: Philosophical Issues / 73
DAVID F. HULTSCH AND JANE H. MCEWAN

7 The Calculus of Discrimination: Discriminatory Resource Allocation for an Aging Population / 84
EIKE-HENNER W. KLUGE

8 Population Aging and the Economy: Some Issues in Resource Allocation / 98
FRANK T. DENTON AND BYRON G. SPENCER

PART TWO: SPECIFIC ISSUES

9 The Right to Participate: Ending Discrimination Against the Elderly / 127
DONALD J. MACDOUGALL

10 Society and Essentials for Well-Being: Social Policy and the Provision of Care / 142
NEENA L. CHAPPELL

11 Foregoing Treatment: Killing versus Letting Die, and the Issue of Non-Feeding / 155
EARL R. WINKLER

12 Foregoing Life-Sustaining Treatment: The Canadian Law Reform Commission and the President's Commission / 172
ALISTER BROWNE

13 Proxy Consent for Research on the Incompetent Elderly / 183
BARRY F. BROWN

14 Gerontology's Challenge from Its Research Population / 194
BEVERLY BURNSIDE

15 Civil Liberties and the Elderly Patient / 208
ARTHUR SCHAFER

16 Narrative, Perspective, and Aging / 215
C.G. PRADO

PART THREE

Bibliography / 225
JAMES E. THORNTON, ANNE D. EVANS, MEGAN STUART-STUBBS, GERRY BATES

General Index / 247
Index of Names / 253

ACKNOWLEDGMENTS

In 1980, the Committee on Gerontology at the University of British Columbia instituted a program of interdisciplinary work with the aim of studying the experiences of aging people and the issues of aging in society. It has undertaken activities which explore "world views" and differing conceptions of aging and being old. Many of the papers in this volume grew out of a symposium on ethics and aging which the Committee held in 1982; others were invited by the editors in order to widen the scope of this book.

The editors want to acknowledge the work and support of people who were instrumental in bringing this volume to print. First, the conceptual foundation of the volume was developed from the work of a research task group convened by James E. Thornton, Co-ordinator, Committee on Gerontology, during 1983 and 1984. Its members at the University of British Columbia included Terry R. Anderson, Vancouver School of Theology; Donald J. MacDougall, Faculty of Law; Rose Murakami, School of Nursing; Sydney Segal, Faculty of Medicine; James E. Thornton, Faculty of Education; Earl R. Winkler, Department of Philosophy; and Anne Evans and Gary Kenyo, graduate students in adult education and gerontology.

Finally, the editors gratefully acknowledge Megan Stuart-Stubbs' assistance in reading manuscripts and managing many of the details with authors. The clerical support of Jeannie Young and Bay Gumboc, Faculty of Education, was invaluable to the Committee and editors from 1983 to final publication. The editorial staff at the University of British Columbia Press has provided outstanding advice and encouragement.

Contributors

GERRY MAUD BATES is an M.Ed. student in Adult Education with an interest in Educational Gerontology. She has assisted the UBC Centre for Continuing Education with several Summer Programs for Retired People, and is currently facilitating a poetry group at an adult daycare centre. She recently completed a "Survey of Seniors' Issues" for the Open Learning Agency, Knowledge Network Division.

JOHN C. BENNETT is a Professor and President Emeritus of Union Theological Seminary in New York. He is a minister of the United Church of Christ and is a past president of the American Theological Society and the American Society of Christian Ethics. He has written numerous books on Christianity, politics, and ethics. He is Senior Contributing Editor of *Christianity and Crisis*.

JAMES E. BIRREN is Dean Emeritus of the Andrus Gerontology Center, University of Southern California. Dr Birren is the Brookdale Foundation Distinguished Scholar and a Professor Emeritus of Psychology and Gerontology at the Andrew Norman Institute for Advanced Study on Gerontology and Geriatrics, University of Southern California. He has published over 200 articles on adult development and aging and is perhaps the most widely cited psychologist on those issues. He serves as editor-in-chief of a three-part *Handbook Series on Aging,* the second edition of which was published in 1985, and the third edition of which is being prepared for publication early in the 1990s.

JANE A. BOYAJIAN is the Ombudsman for the State of Washington responsible for designing and monitoring a state-wide complaint resolution system in long-term care; recommending changes in administrative policies and state statutes; public education; and promoting a working relationship with industry, health care providers, state agencies, and advocacy organizations. She is the past Executive Director of the Northwest Institute of Ethics and the Life Sciences and past Director of the Center for the Shaping of Values.

BARRY F. BROWN is an Associate Professor of Philosophy at St Michael's College, University of Toronto. He specializes in metaphysics and ethics, including biomedical ethics. In 1974, he took a clinical residency in medical ethics at the Texas Medical Center in Houston. He is the coordinator of the undergraduate program in Philosophy Applied to the Life Sciences. He serves on the Human Subjects Review Committee at the University of Toronto and is currently the Chairman of the National Board of Directors of the Juvenile Diabetes Foundation—Canada and a trustee of Diabetes Canada. From 1983 to 1986 he was appointed to the Health Research and Development Council of Ontario, advisory to the Minister of Health.

ALISTER BROWNE teaches philosophy at the Langara campus of Vancouver Community College, and is Vice-President of the BC Civil Liberties Association. His current field of interest and specialization is biomedical ethics, and he has published in the areas of experimentation, death, euthanasia, and abortion.

BEVERLY BURNSIDE received her PH.D. degree in anthropology from the University of Washington in 1977. She holds an honorary research associate appointment in the Department of Health Care and Epidemiology and the Faculty of Graduate Studies' Committee on Gerontology at the University of British Columbia. Dr Burnside pursues social research while conducting community action programs relating to the role of social environmental factors in health/illness among older adults. Ethical issues arising from these activities prompted her involvement in formulating Ethical Guidelines for the Society for Applied Anthropology in Canada during 1983–4.

NEENA L. CHAPPELL has a PH.D. in sociology. She is founding Director of the research Centre on Aging at the University of Manitoba and a National Health Scholar. She has conducted research for several years in the area of informal and formal support systems, health, and health care of the aging. She has published extensively in this area, including two books: Chappell, N.L., Strain, L.A., and Blandford, A.A., *Aging and Health Care: A Social Perspective*. Toronto: Holt, Rinehart and Winston 1986; and Driedger, L. and Chappell, N.L., *Aging and Ethnicity: Toward an Interface*. Toronto: Butterworths 1987.

FRANK I. DENTON is Professor of Economics and Director of the Program for Quantitative Studies in Economics and Population at McMaster University. He has held various positions in government and industry, including several years with Statistics Canada. He is an elected member of the International Statistical Institute and the International Union of the Scientific

Study of Population. He is also a Fellow of the American Statistical Association and of the Royal Society of Canada. He has published extensively in the areas of quantitative economics, population economics, and labour force analysis.

ANNE D. EVANS, B.Sc. (Nursing), M.Ed., is the Corporate Service Advisor for the Registered Nurses' Association of British Columbia and has written a course in Ethics and the Health Sciences for the British Columbia Institute of Technology. She has done extensive bibliographic research on ethical issues and health care of the elderly.

DAVID F. HULTSCH is Lansdowne Professor of Psychology at the University of Victoria. His research is focused primarily on memory and cognitive development during adulthood and aging. Recent publications include: Hultsch, D.F., Hertzog, C., Dixon, R.A., & Davidson, H. (1988). Memory self-knowledge and self-efficacy in the aged. In M.L. Howe & C.J. Brainerd (Eds), *Cognitive development in adulthood: Progress in cognitive development research*. New York: Springer-Verlag; and Hultsch, D.F., Hertzog, C., & Dixon, R.A. (1987). Age differences in metamemory: Resolving the inconsistencies. *Canadian Journal of Psychology*, 41, 193–208. In addition to over 40 articles and chapters, Dr Hultsch has co-authored introductory texts on adult development and aging and developmental psychology.

EIKE-HENNER W. KLUGE teaches at the University of Victoria, specializing in medical ethics of resource allocation, codes of ethics, and proxy decision-making. His publications include *The Practice of Death, The Ethics of Deliberate Death, Withholding Treatment from Defective Newborn Children* (co-authored with J. Magnet), and various articles in the *CMAJ, BCMJ, Canadian Nurse, Theoretical Medicine,* and the *Dalhousie Law Journal*. He is a member of the Ethics Advisory Panel of the BC Ministry of Health, and the first expert witness in medical ethics in a Canadian court of law.

DONALD J. MACDOUGALL is a Professor of Law at the University of British Columbia. He is Vice-President of the International Society on Family Law and Managing Editor, *Canadian Journal of Family Law*. Dr MacDougall's special interests are the constitutional division of legislative power in family law; economic rights within the family; children and the law; the law and the elderly; and alternatives to judicial resolutions of disputes. A recent article on "Working, Learning and Living" appeared in *An Older Workforce: Legal Aspects and Policy Implications,* Occasional Paper No 28, Centre for Human Settlements, University of British Columbia.

JANE H. MCEWAN is a psychologist, and has several years of experience in providing counselling and clinical services within the health care system. Currently she is a PH.D. candidate at the University of Victoria. Her research interests include personality factors and social-environmental variables which influence adult development, and the maintenance of cognitive functioning in later life.

C.G. PRADO is a Professor of Philosophy at Queen's University, Kingston, and author of *The Limits of Pragmatism, Rethinking How We Age: A New View of the Aging Mind, Making Believe: Philosophical Reflections on Fiction,* and *Illusions of Faith: A Critique of Noncredal Religion,* as well as various articles that have appeared in *Nous, Dialogue,* and the *Australasian Journal of Philosophy.*

DAVID ROY is the founder and director of the Center for Bioethics, Clinical Institute of Montreal. He is research professor in the Department of Medicine at the Université de Montréal and has co-ordinated and taught courses in medical ethics and jurisprudence in the medical schools of McGill University in Montreal and the Université Laval in Quebec City. Dr Roy holds degrees in mathematics, philosophy, and theology. He earned his PH.D. (summa cum laude) from the Westfälische Wilhelms Universität, Münster, West Germany, in 1972. He was one of Canada's three official representatives to the Summit Nations International Meetings on Bioethics. He is part of a Working Group set up by the Royal Society of Canada to assess the impact of AIDS on Canadians and he also sits on the newly formed Working Group on AIDS set up by the Ministry of Social Affairs of the Quebec government. He has lectured and published extensively, and serves as consultant on ethical issues dealing with aging and Alzheimer's disease.

ARTHUR SCHAFER is Director of the Centre for Professional and Applied Ethics at the University of Manitoba. He is also the Head of the Section of Bio-Medical Ethics in the Faculty of Medicine, and a Full Professor in the Department of Philosophy. Part of his work as an ethics consultant involves case discussions with physicians and other health care professionals when particularly troubling dilemmas arise in a hospital setting. Professor Schafer has published widely (in philosophical, medical, and legal journals) in moral, social, and political philosophy. He writes on topics to do with biomedical ethics for *The Globe and Mail,* and is a frequent contributor to CBC radio and television.

BYRON G. SPENCER is a Professor of Economics and a Research Associate in the Program for Quantitative Studies in Economics and Population at McMaster University. He is an Elected Member of the International Union for the Scientific Study of Population. He has published extensively in population economics as well as in labour economics and applied econometrics.

CANDACE A. STACEY, PH.D., is a Postdoctoral Fellow in the Department of Psychology at the University of Southern California and a Clinical Geropsychologist at the university-affiliated Andrus Older Adult Center, a research, training, and service center for mental health problems of older adults. She was awarded a Social Science and Humanities Research Council of Canada Predoctoral Fellowship, a National Institute on Aging Predoctoral Training Grant, and a National Institute of Mental Health Postdoctoral Fellowship. Her research interests inlcude psychological well-being among older adults, exercise and aging, housing for the elderly, and neuropsychological assessment.

MEGAN STUART-STUBBS is an MA student in Adult Education at the University of British Columbia. Her interests are in learning over the lifespan, cooperative learning experiences, and ethical considerations in the provision of education.

JAMES E. THORNTON, PH.D., is Coordinator of the Committee on Gerontology, Faculty of Graduate Studies at the University of British Columbia. He teaches Adult Education (Educational Gerontology) in the Department of Administrative, Adult and Higher Education, Faculty of Education. He received his PH.D. in Adult Education from the University of Michigan. In 1984–5 Dr Thornton was a Faculty Fellow, Andrew Norman Institute for Advanced Studies in Gerontology and Geriatrics, Andrus Gerontology Center, University of Southern California, and Visiting Research Scholar in educational gerontology at the Department of Geriatric and Long Term Care Medicine, University of Gothenberg, Sweden, and Department of Adult Education and Social Education, Kyoto University, Japan. His research interests concern the impact of educational and social programs on the well-being of the elderly.

EARL R. WINKLER is Associate Professor of Philosophy at the University of British Columbia. His major areas of interest include theoretical ethics; practical ethics, especially biomedical ethics; philosophy of mind; social and political philosophy; and philosophy and literature. Articles of his have appeared in journals in the United States, Canada, and England, with recent publications being mainly in theoretical ethics and biomedical ethics. He frequently appears on radio and television in connection with issues in biomedical ethics. Current work in progress includes a book on *Foregoing Life-Sustaining Treatments* and one on ethical theory.

Ethics and Aging

1

Introduction to Principal Themes and Issues

EARL R. WINKLER AND JAMES E. THORNTON

The age distribution in North America has begun to shift significantly toward increasing numbers of elderly people in the general population. This trend is expected to combine with general economic limitations to impose further strains and pressures on social institutions and health care delivery systems. Accordingly, a significant body of literature, dominated by demographic and sociological issues, has recently emerged on the complex problems of providing health care and other services for the aged. In general, the ethical dimensions of social policy decisions concerning the elderly have received relatively little attention. Yet the question of the place and claims of the elderly in society is pre-eminently a moral one. Questions about the rights of the elderly to various kinds of social services, about the allocation of health care resources for the elderly, about the forms of professional service society is obligated to provide, and about the responsibilities the elderly are expected to assume are all primarily moral issues.

THE RELEVANCE OF ETHICS TO AGING

In the most general sense, the moral question regarding any action or policy is always "What ought to be done, all things considered?" Because *all* things are considered, moral argument and assessment, moral reasoning, and justification should not be seen as kinds of reasoning which stand in opposition to economic or other "practical" reasons. Moral reasoning and justification, properly understood, are not comparable to, and do not compete with, other distinct modes of reasoning about matters of policy and conduct. The moral point of view is comprehensive and practical in that it takes in all considerations which are relevant to the rational determination of any important issue of policy or practice.

However, the phrase "moral reasons" may legitimately refer to those reasons which predominantly or characteristically come into play in moral discourse and argument – reasons of right and justice, reasons of overall benefit or of legitimate claim and expectation, and utilitarian reasons focusing on general human welfare. Obviously, the issues of public policy and professional practice concerning the role, functioning, treatment, and welfare of the elderly are essentially problems of social morality and have many facets and dimensions. From this perspective, the relevance of ethics to an analysis and exploration of these practical moral issues is straightforward. For insofar as ethics differs from morality, it involves a theoretical and systematically organized investigation of the basic concepts, values, and principles which guide or ought to guide processes of moral decision. Theoretical ethics centrally utilizes analytic resources, such as the clarification of important distinctions, the conceptual exploration of the limits of various principles and of possible conflicts between them, and so forth. Applied ethics tries to interpret and apply basic values and principles in the detailed investigation and resolution of moral issues within some restricted field of social practice, such as medicine, social welfare policy, scientific research, international business, or nuclear defence.

Yet the relations between normative and practical ethics is by no means unidirectional. The recent orientation of ethics toward the complex realities of practical domains has profoundly influenced contemporary currents in ethical theory. This confrontation with the ambiguities of moral reality has led, for example, to important reinterpretations of certain basic ideas and principles, such as the ideal of the "sanctity of human life"; it has led generally to a deepened sense of the fundamental nature of some forms of moral conflict; and it has frequently given rise to a chastened awareness of the tensions inherent in all deep and interesting moral problems, with consequent efforts to accommodate this awareness in theories about the nature and limits of moral reasoning and knowledge. These complications in the relations between theoretical and applied ethics notwithstanding, inasmuch as clarity, rigour, and rational order are valuable, it surely must be clear how important, and even essential, ethics in a comprehensive form must be to the complex process of coming to terms with the various issues concerning aging and the aged.

CENTRAL ISSUES

For a variety of historical and cultural reasons, we presently confront a vast array of practical moral problems and decisions concerning the status, role, and welfare of the elderly in society. Concerning large-scale determinants of the present situation, one thinks of the breakdown of the extended family, increasing population mobility, the institution of old-age security and pension plans, the effect of near-universal retirement, the expansion of technological means of sustaining life, and, most immediately, the prominence of current general concerns with individual rights and claims – to autonomy, health care, equality, and so forth. Besides understanding their historical origins, the problems resulting from these causes must also be considered in the light of changing demographics, which indicate a continuing increase in the percentage of elderly in the population well into the twenty-first century.

To begin with a general problem: what are our culturally most prominent, pervasive, and influential attitudes and beliefs about aging, particularly as regards ideas about decline, dependency, productive or contributory potential, and proper place and function? In what ways might any of these ideas and attitudes be inappropriate, dysfunctional, or maladaptive for the individual or the general good of society? Is it true, for instance, as some have charged, that because of our dominant concern with material and consumer values and the resulting primary orientation toward the generation currently holding power and exercising authority, we tend, in our thoughts about aging, to be overly dominated by ideas and fears of decline and dependency? After all, through a strenuously competitive and materialistic social organization, we do put a premium on independence and power, so it should not be surprising if we tend to make thoughts about their diminution and loss central to our understanding and anticipation of aging. One wonders how much this socio-psychological phenomenon has contributed to what is now generally recognized as an unfortunate tendency to overly medicalize, segregate, and institutionalize the care of the aged. As William May notes,[1] by segregating the exigent and the aged into the care of competent professionals, we protect ourselves from reminders of our own vulnerability and our own fear, at the same time converting the occasion into one in which the dominant community exhibits its precedence and power. In any case, it is both clear and somewhat surprising, in light of economic factors alone, that we provide too few alternatives for the elderly intermediate between life in a family setting, or complete independence, and complete institutional care. Yet what mix of intermediate programs should be provided, and with what priorities?

From another angle, one can ask to what extent culturally dominant attitudes and beliefs about aging have biased the forms and styles of research on aging, and even the very forms of ethical discourse about aging itself. Both research and moral discourse have tended to treat the elderly in decidedly passive ways, as subjects upon whom to investigate and experiment and for whom to do various things. Neither science nor morals has evinced much regard for what the elderly themselves might actively contribute to research direction and design or to planning and implementation of social policy, or much concern with what might legitimately be expected from the elderly in society. This pervasive condescension by the intellectual community reduces the aged to moral nonentities.[2]

Consider next the way in which various questions of conceptual analysis, and questions of the rational adjudication between competing or conflicting values, arise in connection with the application of certain fundamental concepts, such as "autonomy," "paternalism," "competence," "rationality," "informed consent," and so forth. For example, might there be cases in which an elderly patient's refusal of treatment is legally competent but is also judged to be sufficiently irrational to justify intervention in the patient's own interests? More generally, does a principle of autonomy in decisionmaking merely require competency, as usually understood, or is a stronger condition required, like rational coherence with the patient's own most important values? In short, how are we to balance the sometimes conflicting claims of individual autonomy and sound humanitarian practice?

Other issues, occurring primarily in clinical contexts, are more prominent in the public consciousness but hardly nearer resolution. Consider, for example, the question of what moral and legal authority should be accorded so-called "living wills." There is also the very common problem of what conditions ethically justify or permit the withdrawal of certain treatments which only serve to prolong a life without human meaning or dignity. This, of course, in its turn raises the question of whether there is any genuine and morally relevant distinction between passive and active euthanasia, that is, between allowing someone to die and deliberately bringing about his or her death for reasons of mercy. Also significant, regarding alternatives in dealing with death and dying, is the current hospice movement with its claims to social, economic, and individual advantage. Finally, throughout the entire range of moral decisions concerning the treatment of the aged in clinical settings, there looms the question of *who* should decide these matters when patients themselves cannot, particularly whether the decision belongs primarily with patients' families or with physicians.

There is also concern regarding both general standards of professionalism and research on the aged. How does the quality of service provided in our society by professionals dealing with the elderly compare with the quality of care and service provided to younger, more energetic and powerful groups? Moreover, the aged, particularly those in large public clinics, are especially vulnerable to various forms of experimentation that are easily integrated with standard therapy, in which principles of informed consent are remarkably relaxed. These and similar issues need to be raised and discussed in the interests of professional self-regulation, improvement and accountability.

An especially difficult general issue is that of social justice in the distribution of health care resources to various subgroups within the population. What principles and procedures ought to govern this matter of allocation of scarce resources?

Lastly, one should consider a very important problem concerning the social role and position of the elderly. The issue is that of fair and appropriate public policy on retirement and pensions. Contrary economic and social pressures conspire to produce a genuine dilemma. On the one hand, because of the increasing economic strains on public financing of retirement and entitlement programs, there is increased pressure on the elderly to remain at work as long as they are able, out of self-interest and to avoid dependency or becoming a burden. On the other hand, the continuing problem of unemployment creates an opposite pressure for them to retire and make room for younger or more needy persons to enter the work force. While the elderly continue to be generally subject to either neglect or sometimes overtreatment, these opposing pressures are likely to make them subject to resentment as well, regarded as a threat either because they are working or because they are not.

ORIENTATION OF THIS BOOK

The overall aim of this collection of papers is to contribute to two recent trends in the field of ethics and gerontology. First and more generally, this anthology represents a thoroughly interdisciplinary approach to the ethical dimensions of social and health policy concerning aging. The field of biomedical ethics has become increasingly desegregated and interdisciplinary in recent years. This approach is producing some shared professional vocabulary and a shared appreciation of the real complexity of many of its issues, particularly those with the potential for genuine conflict among basic values. All must agree that the moral problems concerning aging have many irreducible facets. Accurate understanding and judicious response, therefore, demand some integration of the experience, sensibility, and knowledge provided by different professional and scientific perspectives. Viewpoints from theology, philosophy, sociology, psychology, gerontology, medicine, nursing, economics, and law are all represented here, often directed toward similar or related issues. The drawbacks of this interdisciplinary approach – in terms of discursive untidiness, the absence of a unified voice and perspective, and the presence of varying conceptions of ethics – are offset by the advantage, important at this juncture, of being able to see and compare different professional treatments of some of the basic moral problems concerning aging. This approach, moreover, has the overriding virtue of providing the opportunity for a more comprehensive appreciation of the relevant moral issues than could be achieved by attempting to treat them as the province of a single specialty, especially that of general, theoretical ethics.

The second development in ethics and gerontology to which this book is directed is more particular but less consolidated, and hence, at this point, more significant. It concerns the involvement of the elderly in the ethical and scientific community as individuals with ideas, values, virtues, standards, and responsibilities of their own. A large majority of the papers collected here are united in giving central place in their arguments to considerations regarding the dignity of the person. In one form or another, these papers reflect the centrality of ideas of autonomy, dignity, and personal responsibility, and of rights and obligations deriving from these concepts. Accordingly, many of these papers speak, in different ways, of social, psychological, and procedural obstacles that reduce the humanity of the elderly, both in daily life and in institutional settings. Some pieces explicitly emphasize the need for various practical reforms that will enhance the direct participation of the elderly in the social and scientific processes that are directed toward them. In others, considerable stress is given to the importance of recognizing the elderly as bearers of certain responsibilities as well as rights, thus taking them seriously as moral agents and not merely as dependent subjects of social policy, however benevolently motivated such policy might be.

Thus, beneath the diversity of topics and points of view represented in this volume, there exists a general orientation toward a common moral centre of gravity. It is this general, thematic orientation toward the dignity of the person that may be expected to contribute to the growing concern for the fullest recognition of the humanity of the elderly.

ORGANIZATION OF THE PAPERS

The papers are divided into two main groups. Papers in the first group are of two kinds. Some provide a general perspective on various ethical issues involving the aged – for example, defining the main moral problems arising in a given context, such as clinical medicine or research with the aged – while others provide background information of a conceptual or empirical form, such as models of aging or of demographic trends, which are essential to identifying and assessing ethical issues. Papers in the second group each define and explore – and sometimes attempt to resolve – a specific issue of moral importance related to aging and the elderly, such as the moral fairness of mandatory retirement, or the adequacy of the present structure of health care, or participation by the elderly in public policy and research.

It may be helpful at this point to briefly describe the main themes of each of the papers and to indicate some important relations between them.

Jane A. Boyajian offers a humanitarian introduction to many of the issues we confront in our treatment of and provision for the aged. Her concern is with the human complexity and ambiguity of our relations with them, both in clinical and geriatric settings and beyond. There are, for example, the disturbing gap between our aspirations and the reality of the services we provide; the problem of balancing the need for efficiency and cost-effectiveness with the moral demand to recognize and support individuality and autonomy; the frustrating difficulty of determining competence for self-decisions in individual cases; the complications of motive in many of our decisions, whether we act to protect ourselves or in the true interests of the aged person; the problem of fairness in the allocation of scarce resources.

David Roy deepens our understanding of the many issues concerning aging that arise in clinical settings. Reflecting first on the dangers of biased attitudes toward the aged, he goes on to consider what we may expect over the next quarter-century concerning increasing numbers of elderly people and their health care needs. He draws attention to the ways these changes may affect the already prominent and controversial issues concerning death and dying in the clinical setting. In this connection, Roy first gives us a robust rejection of cost-benefit analysis in determining issues of resource allocation for the aged. He then proceeds to a fuller discussion of the topics of dignity in death and of passive and active euthanasia.

John C. Bennett (himself an octogenarian) provides a personal perspective focusing on several fundamental values which he believes should guide our efforts and relations with the elderly. The values themselves are familiar, those of justice, freedom, and responsibility. These are discussed and interrelated in the context of many everyday topics and examples. Of particular interest is the stress Bennett lays on the need to recognize the elderly as autonomous beings with responsibilities as well as rights. He closes his paper with a balanced presentation of the issue of active assistance in death for certain cases.

James E. Birren and Candace A. Stacy briefly review the scientific literature concerning the aging process, particularly regarding alternative perspectives of growth versus decline during the course of life. Though the evidence is complex and ambiguous, they conclude that science indicates roughly that aging involves a decline along some dimensions of performance and functioning and growth in others. This requires that we seek metaphors of aging that are capable of reflecting this tension between growth and decline. They argue that we have an obligation to both ourselves and others to continually evaluate, upgrade, and improve our conception and models of aging in light of scientific findings and more extensive human understanding. One of the most compelling features of aging is the human organism's ability to actively compensate for various declining capacities. And, most importantly, Birren and Stacy point out that how we regard ourselves, our very self-concepts and their associated expectations, are themselves partially self-determining.

More generally noteworthy is the fact that this paper is informed by a pre-enlightenment conception of moral philosophy having affinities with an Aristotelian concern for the basic conditions of a good or well-lived life. Thomas Cole has recently suggested that a renewal of this ancient cultural conversation about the conditions of a good life will prove necessary to adequately understand and manage the moral problems of aging.[3] For it is from this cultural conversation that we develop inwardly compelling ideas about the ends of human life, without which aging must always in some measure be feared.

The normative complexity of scientific intervention in the aging process is analysed by David Hultsch and Jane H. McEwan. First, the intervention process is itself a complex set of decisions involving various normative evaluations or assumptions. For example, simply to see the elderly as suffering certain deficits relative to the performance skills of younger groups and then to try to alleviate this condition is to assume the behaviour of young adults as the criterion of optimum functioning. Moreover, the goals of the clientele, viz. the aged, are rarely considered or given prominent place in the development of intervention programs. Second, Hultsch and McEwan argue that we must recognize more fully that intervention represents an intrusion into an entire system of interrelated components. They offer various illustrations of the pitfalls of failing to adequately appreciate these functional interrelationships prior to intervention.

Eike-Henner W. Kluge takes up the general issue of justice and fairness in the allocation of health care resources when these are limited. Following a rejection of cost-benefit and cost-effectiveness theories, he offers a schematic rights-based framework for considering issues of allocation and draws certain conclusions regarding its relevance for health care policies concerning the elderly. Since the position Kluge takes is a general one, there are various connections between his paper and some of the others. For example, consider the link with Neena L. Chappell's analysis of the Canadian health care system. Partly on behalf of the elderly, Chappell argues for a generally more expansive and more flexible system of health care. Many of the alternative services she envisages, such as various forms of home care, would be of special relevance to the aged. In this connection, Kluge's paper offers a theoretical framework for fairly considering the claims of the elderly for special allocations of health care resources against the competing claims of other groups.

In her paper, Chappell offers a brief historical sketch of the development of the Canadian health care system. She criticizes its current structure as being restrictively dominated by a medical model of health and illness. The medical model brings with it an overemphasis on the services of physicians and on institutional care. Chappell argues that the present health care system requires restructuring to achieve a generally greater flexibility in providing alternatives to exclusively physician-controlled treatment and institutionalized care, including more social and community services, more chronic and home care services, and the like. She sees these developments as necessary to the promotion of dignity and autonomy for the aged.

Frank T. Denton and Byron G. Spencer do not define or discuss any specifically ethical issues related to aging. Rather, they provide a very important analysis of the overall population aging process and its probable effect on different sectors of the Canadian economy over the next several decades. Of particular relevance to the ethical issue of fair and just allocation of public resources for the aged, however, is their central claim that overall dependency ratios in the Canadian population as it ages over the course of the next half century will not be excessive by historical standards. Denton and Spencer argue that the increased proportion of dependent elderly will be offset in large measure by smaller proportions of dependent children and higher proportions of people of working age. According to these projections, our main social and moral problems arising from the aging of the population will have much more to do with the reallocation of resources than with an insufficiency of total resources to meet changing demands.

From a legal perspective on allocation and equity, Donald J. MacDougall is concerned with the ethical conflicts which can arise between the claims of the individual and those of society, most frequently in the form of a tension between individual rights and social utility. He develops the issues of age discrimination, income security for the aged, and compulsory retirement as concrete examples of this kind of ethical conflict. The central questions are whether compulsory retirement policies involve unjustifiable age discrimination and to what extent society is obligated to provide adequate financial security for the aged.

Earl R. Winkler's paper addresses the issue of active and passive euthanasia, which is discussed cursorily by Roy and more personally by Bennett. Winkler first analyses the moral relevance of the killing/letting die distinction and then considers the controversial issue of the morality of withholding foods and fluids.

Going beyond the specific concerns raised by Winkler, Alister Browne continues the discussion of cessation of treatment and related issues. First he compares and evaluates the central recommendations of recent Canadian and United States commission reports on these matters. He then concentrates on the crucial question of *who* is to decide for incompetent patients. In pursuing this question, Browne offers arguments concerning the proper office of ethics committees and the usefulness of advance declarations or "living wills."

Barry F. Brown is concerned with the issue of experimentation on the incompetent elderly. Can this be justified through proxy consent in non-therapeutic contexts, for example with Alzheimer's disease? Brown shows that current interpretations of several basic principles of biomedical ethics, particularly the principles of benevolence and respect for persons, leave this issue unresolved. These principles put the interests or claims of the individual in stark tension with those of society at large. Through a comparison with an earlier debate over experimentation on non-consensual children, Brown seeks a revised conception of the common good, one which reduces the conflict between the social good and that of the individual.

The issue of the democratization of research on the aged is taken up by Beverly Burnside. She perceives a need for consultation between researchers and the elderly as research subjects. In various forms, provision should be made for collaboration on the definition of problems, on research goals and design, and on interpretation of findings. In making her case, Burnside compares the present situation in gerontology with an earlier one in which anthropology faced a similar challenge.

According to Arthur Schafer, elderly patients are frequently subjected to unjustifiable restraint and deprivation of liberty. He believes that much of this abuse derives from the prevalence of an inappropriate paternalistic model of care employed by medical staff and family. Using case analysis, Schafer challenges the moral legitimacy of this model by contrasting it with a competing civil liberties model.

C.G. Prado begins with a recognition of prejudice in widespread attitudes toward aging. He believes that the essence of this prejudicial attitude comes from a presumption of increasing narrow-mindedness, or perspective narrowing, as a direct function of aging. In an effort to defeat this presumption of serious decline in adaptive competency with aging, Prado seeks a reinterpretation of changes in mental functioning that are characteristic of aging. He sees certain of these changes as the effect not of deterioration but of adaptive functions naturally leading to greater (and sometimes too great) interpretive parsimony in processing the data of experience. Prado's paper provides an interesting contribution to the general discussion of growth versus decline with aging and the ethical dimensions of our beliefs and attitudes in this area.

The contributors to this book have no common discipline, doctrinal perspective, or theory of value. Although the papers share overlapping problems and themes, the variability in points of view, styles of argument, and specific proposals testifies to the complexity of the broad domain addressed by the book as a whole. As we confront the social challenge of dealing with the many problems posed by an aging population, we urgently require a deeper appreciation of the ethical dimensions of our policies and undertakings. This book represents a modest but, we hope, significant contribution toward this deepened awareness. It will be useful to professionals and practitioners in the health care field, to gerontologists and sociologists, to those who study and teach in the area of biomedical ethics, to hospital administrators, public policy analysts, and to lawyers and legislators concerned with the formation of social policy affecting the aged.[4]

NOTES

1 William May, *Hastings Center Report,* vol. 12, no. 6 (Hastings-on-Hudson, NY: Institute of Society, Ethics and Life Sciences 1983)

2 William May, ''The Virtues and Vices of the Elderly,'' in Thomas R. Cole and Sally A. Gadow, eds., *What Does It Mean to Grow Old?* (Durham: Duke University Press 1986), 43

3 Thomas R. Cole, ''Aging and Meaning,'' *Generations* (Winter 1985), 51

4 The editors wish to acknowledge having benefited from referees' comments on earlier drafts of this introduction as well as from their suggestions for revising the papers.

PART ONE

General Perspectives

2

On Reaching a New Agenda: Self-Determination and Aging

JANE A. BOYAJIAN

I ask the reader to consider words that professionals who serve the elderly use daily, such as "basic science," "autonomy," and "freedom." My purpose is to reflect on the intrinsic meaning of these words, away from the bureaucratic policies and procedures which shape our work as professionals, and to ask: what underlying principles should we, as morally sensitive professionals, bear in mind as we promote policies and develop services for elders? What are the visions which first drew us to our work? Because this paper primarily addresses ethical issues, it is written in the language of ethics.

The section "On Subtleties" reviews basic issues in ethical analysis as they pertain to elders. It invites the reader to reflect on the more subtle aspects of our policies and procedures, and reminds the reader of the importance of separating personal values from professional decisionmaking. "On Balance" reconsiders autonomy, freedom, cost-benefit analysis, equity, and efficiency from the perspective of ethics rather than those of social science research or law. The importance of promoting the elderly's continuing participation in life rather than allowing them to become marginalized is then discussed. The final section, "On Well-Being," asks the reader to push beyond legal and procedural terms. Well-being is here redefined – it is more than freedom to be self-determining. An individual experiences well-being when she/he can thrive in the fullest sense of that word, becoming all that she/he can be despite age, illness, and financial circumstances.

My concern – and yours – is our elders. These are the women and men who gave us life, who have been our models. Their realities created our yesterdays, and their dreams still shape our tomorrows. Because we are concerned here with ethics and aging, you and I are concerned with doing good. For us this means providing elders with what they need, especially when they can no longer get those essentials for themselves. So we work hard to ensure that they have the basics (food, shelter, warmth) even when resources shrink.

As we focus our attention on the ethical aspects of caring for elders, we concern ourselves with their well-being. By this I mean more than seeing that our elders are fed, more than keeping our social welfare system intact to provide for them when they are sick. Of course, food, shelter, clothing, and medical services are essential. But we are also concerned about the conditions in which the elderly can thrive. We are talking about much more than simply providing what is needed for physical survival. As reflective and sensitive people, we know that food can fill bellies yet not nourish; that food can nourish yet not satisfy. We know that clothing and housing may keep one warm and dry, yet not sustain the spirit. And we are abundantly aware that providing for illness is not the same as promoting health.

Recognizing these distinctions is a step toward an awareness of what elders essentially need and of what our responsibilities as care providers should be. Unfortunately, the programs and services we deliver to our elders do not take into account these distinctions. There is usually a great gap between what our elders really need and want and what we are actually willing to provide them.

Our services tell us a great deal, and the lack of services, which impede or damage well-being, also proclaim our values. After all, what we do for one another, and how we do it, is an expression of what we value. Often the services we provide reflect only what we think the elderly need. (Do we ever ask them directly?) Sometimes, our service delivery serves only to justify our own existence as service providers. Often we forget that that which sustains and nourishes the spirit is at least as important as clothing and bread.

ON SUBTLETIES

We must pay attention to subtleties. Making choices is never simple. And when we make personal, social, institutional, and public policy choices for those who are vulnerable and, therefore, dependent upon our goodwill, our choicemaking is even more complex. Choosing responsibly what services we should provide elders means first examining and untangling our own motives. We should ask ourselves, "Why do we think we know what is 'best' for them?"

Choosing responsibly requires, secondly, that we listen to the recipients of our services. What do they say they need? What do they say they fear? What do they want, as opposed to what we think they need? Furthermore, we must find the delicate balance between doing things for others to provide them with the basics that they cannot themselves supply and respecting them as persons. We are often confused about this: we seem unaware of the fine line between caring for others respectfully and taking away their sense of personhood, their distinctiveness as individuals. Current discussions about the difference between self-neglect and personal idiosyncracies in life style begin to acknowledge these subtleties.

Ethical decisionmaking in our professional practice often involves a difficult balancing act, in which we must juggle several goods we value. And ethical sensitivity requires attentiveness to subtleties – being able to discern what values we express by our actions. As we reflect, we can see that decisions which initially seemed to be straightforward may actually be quite complex. Issues which at first seemed important fade as others suddenly come into view. Subtleties emerge.

The nature of an ethical dilemma is having to choose between several goods we value when we cannot serve all. So we must reflect upon what is at stake; the goals (ends) we would achieve and the methods (means) by which we would achieve them must be examined. For example, two principles traditionally guide physicians' decisions regarding their patients: to do no harm and to bring aid. These principles have always seemed straightforward tools for decisionmaking: always seek not to hurt but to help. Yet in the previous three decades, medical practice had changed so much that by the early 1970s physicians could see that some interventions they had used with the intention of helping patients actually caused some of them harm by prolonging a painful dying process. Probing actions and consequences, evaluating intentions and values, and exploring subtleties gained new importance.

ON DYING

The case of dying may help to illustrate what I mean by attending to subtleties. There is much discussion now of the rights of the dying and of our responsibility to those who are dying. We have slowly come to see that in our providing for others in the institutional setting we have sometimes forgotten that it is *someone else's body* for whom we are providing. However well-intentioned our motives, we have usurped the right of patients or clients to choose what should (or should not) happen to their bodies. In the last decade, we have gradually become clearer about to whom such decisions actually belong – the patients themselves. In addition, awareness and concern for our legal liability have caused us to examine how we provide for others. We have been forced to re-examine our assumption that we as professionals know what is best for others. We have even begun to acknowledge that our own motives in deciding for others are not always clear or pure: that is, our motives really reflect what *we* want. Thus, what we say often merely suits our goals for care, teaching, or research. With greater awareness about patient rights and misuse of professional power, most of us now recognize that decisions about care, even at the end of life, rest with the patient. As a result, we are beginning to review our practice as professionals. Some papers in this volume illustrate that process of sorting out our own values from patient wishes.

Ethical reflection has greatly shaped this re-examination. For it is also true that we are becoming more ethically sophisticated – aware of the subtleties in our decisions. We recognize more and more the importance of attending to both the universal and the particular. That is, we can see that decisions about one patient would have broad social and moral implications if we were to treat all cases similarly. We can also see that broad ethical principles and social policies must be mediated by the impact they have on the well-being of real and different people. This means going beyond the obvious.

So we have become more sophisticated about the whole issue of dying and patients' rights – even if we sometimes forget those rights in the daily routines of caring for others. We are at the point in some medical settings of having standardized operating procedures to be employed when a patient requests only comfort care. Gradually, we have developed a common understanding about what constitutes comfort care. Generally speaking, giving comfort care means no heroics or interventions which only prolong the dying process. It means caring for the patient respectfully, providing all which one realistically can for that patient's comfort during the dying – warmth, cleanliness, freedom from pain.

Now, new questions emerge. For example, we understand that a patient's request for "no tubes" means no respirator or nasogastric tubes. But does it mean no nourishment or liquids by intravenous feeding? When do these provide comfort to the dying person so that we would want to give them (and the patient would request them if he or she could) even though a secondary effect might be a slower dying process? And when does feeding meet our needs as care providers rather than the patient's?

Recently I was present as a Minneapolis hospital's ethics committee struggled with the issues around artificial feeding and the implications for professional practice. We talked about the artificial nourishment of those unable to tell us what they want: When do we give it? When does it give comfort to the patient? When does it merely comfort us, the care providers? When do our needs fit into the equation? And when is artificial feeding a violation of the person's wish to die naturally? This is what I mean when I say we must attend to subtleties and untangle our motives.

When we discussed whether or not to withdraw artificial feeding, I believe we were talking about more than caloric input. Giving another person food is more than nourishing him or her. The act of giving food is also an act of connection – the connecting of an individual to the community. Theologically speaking, the food becomes the tangible symbol of the community – the embodiment of connectedness – the gift from the community to an individual now distanced from it in every relevant way. Here the giver is the connecting link. The act of giving and receiving becomes a sacramental act.

Our joy in living comes from a sense of our participation in creation – in community. So separation from others – isolation by word, deed, illness, age, or dying – is the epitome of loneliness – aloneness in its most fundamental sense. When I think about ways we can harm others, it seems that banishing them from our community, preventing them from participating to the degree their illnesses permit, is among the greatest transgressions. Conversely, that which affirms connectedness to others is often, though not always, the highest good we can provide. That is really why we continue to talk to the comatose. Seen in this light, feeding a sick or dying person separated from the community can be communion in its broadest, most elemental sense. It can nourish the spirit. Giving food to a dying person who is beyond the more customary ways of interrelating can prolong the dying, possibly against his or her stated wishes, but it can also be a celebration of that person's continuing participation in community, in creation, even while dying.

I do not mean that we should therefore continue feeding dying persons against their wishes. Rather, the example illustrates the subtleties to which I have referred. The real trick for us as care providers is to know whether feeding is actually meeting a patient's needs or meeting our own. If that patient is unable to tell us, how can we know? For we rehearse our own dying when we are with another.

So we can see that giving and receiving services and assessing priorities in human needs can be so complex, so tricky. It is extremely important to push below the surface to examine what is really at stake. The responsible care provider will explore those subtleties.

As I think about nourishing another person in this way, I think how seldom we consider the full meaning of feeding elders who live alone. We talk about the need for meals on wheels, congregate dining, even vitamins – all nutrition for the body. But these are more than merely nutritional programs. They are remembrances from the community. One hopes these programs are respectful and caring of persons. But they are also the tie of connectedness to the community; these programs for our elders are communion with the community and so food for the soul.

If this is the case, we now need to ask: do our programs and outreach really convey this sense of the caring community to elders? Are they respectful of person, of difference? When is what we peevishly call non-compliance (because it upsets our work schedule, our objectives, our values) the expression of our values arbitrarily imposed on others? When we label elders incompetent, might we really mean that we are uncomfortable with their life styles, their decisions? Above all, do our programs and services for elders meet the standard of interaction about which I am speaking here – keeping the individual within the community? If our services are our ways of relating with them, then these programs should be expressions of the joy of connectedness with creation. We must ask ourselves: despite our intentions and our many services to elders, do we miss the mark?

When we think about our elders and their needs, we do them a disservice if we forget that the hard part in caring for another, in showing concern, is paying attention to the subtleties. When we develop public policy and social programs for vulnerable people and fail to examine how those policies affect individual lives and persons who do not precisely fit our bureaucratic categories, we miss the mark. And most of our elders are vulnerable by reason of disability or circumstance.

We need to see elders not as recipients of our programs, though they are, but rather as members of our community-in-the-present. We need to remember that they are separated from our community partly because of their infirmity or living situation but more because of our attitudes toward them. We have placed them at the fringe of existence. We would "do" for them, but in so doing we forget who they are as individuals, and we deny their humanity.

ON BALANCING

We must also become skilful in finding the right balance. As we develop programs for vulnerable people, we must sensitively and reflectively balance several competing goods or values.

Autonomy and protection. We must balance protecting our elders from harm with honouring their autonomy as persons. It is so easy for someone caring for vulnerable persons to slip across the fine line between caring for others and "protecting" them from their own autonomy. Caring for others has to include respecting the person as a unique individual. Respecting a person's autonomy means honouring the choices that person makes about his or her life – remembering that these choices, like our own, flow out of the person's value system and life experiences. It is not our right to "protect" others from their own decisionmaking; otherwise we treat them as objects. So what appears to us to be self-abuse may be to someone else an affirmation of value.

Personal values and medical technology. We must be sensitive to elders' personal values about their care and what, to them, constitutes a life worth living, while at the same time being wary of the quicksand of medical technology. Because we have the technology to extend the living or dying of another, our ability to intervene often fools us into thinking that we ought to do so. We are tempted to do this even when the patient tells us clearly "no more." We are so tempted because we are accustomed to bold interventions in research settings; our definition of success often means a few added months or years, regardless of the patient's quality of life. Sometimes we are tempted to intervene even when patients say no because in their place we would choose otherwise. So we take their naysaying as prima facie evidence of their incompetence. In so doing, we ignore the whole point of informed consent: a voluntary choice is not one which is forced on patients by their care providers. There is no voluntariness when they are permitted only one answer – accepting what the staff say they need. Respecting their decisions means not interfering with their choice even when we think it inappropriate or self-destructive. It means not interfering even though we could get a court order to provide care when they refuse to give consent. We need to remember that sometimes our technologies encourage the preservation of bodies beyond the wishes of patients.

Going beyond cost-benefit analyses. Frankly, we must become both more attentive to the costs of medical care and recognize that the value of a life should not be measured by dollars alone. By this I mean going beyond only cost-benefit analyses. Not considering costs is irresponsible or careless decisionmaking. But so also is basing decisions about the care a patient will receive solely on costs. Of course we as a society must factor in the costs of heart-lung transplants and other crisis interventions when we try to decide who should get our expensive or limited resources. The direct and indirect costs of expensive medical technologies have an important impact upon our medical system and foreclose other possibilities and must be considered in the public arena. But it is inappropriate to make that analysis when we are determining the care plan for a specific patient; at that time, our primary responsibility is what is best for him or her.

Equity. We should strive for equity in health and medical resources while recognizing our special responsibilities to vulnerable groups. This is the issue of fairness. Because our resources are so limited, certain key questions should be before us: How do we decide who gets what care? And when? Surely we do not really mean to triage (choose) based on financial means or proximity to a major medical centre. Yet this is now the basis on which some get care and others do not. And age alone (whether two years or eighty-one) should not be the sole determinant of candidacy for a protocol. Age, costs, and access are pertinent factors in a larger equation – the painful balancing of the needs of one vulnerable group (e.g., elders) against those of another (e.g., children). Accidents of birth should not be the chance determinants of who gets care. Our own conscientious, if painful, decisionmaking should determine this.

Efficiency and responsiveness. We have a responsibility to make our delivery systems more efficient, just as we have a responsibility to make those systems more responsive to persons. Here is a paradox. We must go about the business of doing needs assessments, performing cost-effective discharge planning, and cutting the excess from medical and human services costs. Yet we also need to remember that our elders are persons, not pieces of furniture to be moved periodically or discarded when it suits our notions of fitness, timeliness, neatness, politics, or economy. Efficient procedures must be balanced with responsiveness to the human dimension.

The present and the future. We have a responsibility to future generations even as we honour our continuing covenant with our elders. Both the rapidly growing costs of medical care and the growing recognition that our resources are limited have an impact on our decisionmaking about the care we believe we should provide one another. Just as we must balance the needs of different groups in our society, we must balance our continuing covenant with those who are now a part of our community-of-the-present with our responsibility to the community-of-the-future. Because the future cannot speak for itself, we are its guardians. Of course, we cannot predict with certainty the effects of our present decisions upon it. But responsible decisionmaking calls for conscientious reflection: neither ignoring future impacts nor, out of weakness and sentiment, choosing public policy options today which will unfairly burden future generations. We at least owe our successors the widest possible options. Medical and human service decisions we make now can limit or promote those options. And so we must engage in a complex balancing act indeed – between our desire to do well for the present and our responsibility to the future.

The universal and the personal. Above all, as we struggle with public policy decisions affecting our elders, we need to remember the importance of maintaining a balance between the universal and the personal. Each time we struggle with decisions about the needs and care of one individual, we should also reckon with the public (and, therefore, political) dimensions of that decision. This means asking what values are really driving those decisions. What would happen if we were to treat everyone this way? What kind of a society would we then be creating?

By the same token, as we deliberate about public policy decisions for the many, we need to temper large numbers with the personal. Noting individual life histories and circumstances helps us remember that our choices affect human beings – widely differing individuals. The values and concerns of people vary and arise out of very specific and often painful contexts. If we truly respect persons as individuals, we must pay attention to those particulars. The universal and the personal must go together.

None of these balancing acts is easy. It is hard work finding and sorting out often competing values. Identifying our vested interests and private values as care providers is sometimes a painful struggle. Yet care providers who are ethically alert will recognize the importance of striving to keep clear in their minds that they are serving patient/client needs and values rather than their own.

ON AMBIGUITY

Elders live on the border. They are of us, yet not with us; we have marginalized them, put them at the fringes of our life and awareness. Kafka's Gregor helps us remember how that happens,[1] as we witness his metamorphosis from man to roach.

As Gregor discovers that he is changing into a roach, he tries to behave as he did before the metamorphosis began. Partly this is his denial. His daily routine helps him keep his hold on his sense of personhood, his essential integrity. At the same time, he tries to protect his family from the change which is taking place in his body. "Remaining in his room, Gregor hides from sight whenever anyone enters. . . . He cleans himself regularly, concerns himself with his family's welfare such as he can, and dreaming of freedom, peers from his window."[2]

But, over time, Gregor gives in. The changes he experiences in his body, his new habit of hiding himself from his family, and his isolation from the world outside (since he is now both a curiosity and an object of scorn and hate) all take their toll. His personal hygiene habits unravel. He becomes more roachlike with each day, and his despondency and self-hate grow. He loses his spirit.

At first his relatives, because they are repelled by him, encourage him to keep to his room. But, because they are hopeful, they look for Gregor's return to his earlier state; they continue caring for him as they always have – keeping his room and person clean. Yet they are also horrified at his change. Gradually, they turn their energies and attention elsewhere; he is experienced both as memory of his former self and as burden. Eventually, "hope fades, the reality oppresses, and the family's perception of Gregor changes. . . . The family concludes that the roach was never their son. What is a tragic ending [his death] for the son is a happy ending for the family."[3]

Ronald Preston's reflections on Gregor's story remind us that it has its analogy in the lives of the dying, the aging, and the disabled. Gregor is every person's beloved grandfather. Following a stroke, grandfather's reaction to his illness, as well as the reactions of his family over time, is reminiscent of Gregor. Grandfather and Gregor share a common fate; their abnormality has a fearsome impact upon others. Love turns to scorn, caring becomes duty, affirmation as beloved individual gives way to denial of personhood. Death is a blessing.

The aged and the disabled are ambiguous people. Because they are deviations from the norm, they are regarded with ambivalence by those who love them and care for them; they are taboos. "Taboos are combinations of men and not-men [sic], human and non-human, natural and supernatural; thus they represent the boundaries between these."[4] We are fascinated by their mystery, yet fearful of their meaning for us.

Gregor's and our grandparents' care providers share similar responses: fascination, love at first, avoidance, then distance. These are the common responses of care providers to the ambiguous:

> [She] may rationalize a bridge between [her] definition and the incongruous elements. He may alter his definition so that [which repels] is taken into account. [She] may physically avoid the ambiguous manifestation. . . . He may perceptually avoid manifest ambiguity by concentrating on diversionary interests. [She] may work to remove the ambiguous manifestation and laugh at it to release tension and to persuade [herself] of its inconsequence. He may seek out an ambiguous manifestation so that he may grow inured to it. . . . [She] may rationalize and avoid.[5]

So it can be with those of us who care for the dying, disabled, or aging; Preston's list is a recounting of our own social, political, and institutional responses to aging.

To love and to be loved is to participate in creation, say Dorothee Soelle and Shirley Cloyes.[6] If that is the case, how can we better our programs and services for elders? The food and the rooms we provide and the protocols we develop are only the vehicles through which we nourish others and keep them connected to the community, rather than separated from it.

ON WELL-BEING: A NEW AGENDA

We end where we began. We are concerned here with the ethical and public policy dimensions of our elders' rights and needs. We are concerned with the implications for our own practice as responsible and responsive care providers.

I believe that of course our elders need and have a right to nutrition programs, housekeeping services, and care when they are sick. But more than that, I believe that we should be enhancing the conditions in which they can thrive, as people *can* thrive even when they are sick or dying. What we should be after is their well-being, spiritual and social as well as physical. Until now, most of our attention and meagre financing has been devoted to the physical needs of our elders. Clean, well-fed, and pain-free bodies are important concerns; they should be key priorities. But that simply is not enough! We should be building a new agenda, and the following issues should be central to that agenda.

The Surgeon General of the United States has noted that, while longer life was one of our "most conspicuous accomplishments," our new goal should be "a healthier life for older people."[7] But we must now ask what other factors contribute to well-being? How shall we promote independent, healthy, and rewarding lives for our elders?

The Law Reform Commission of Canada lists two key criteria in defining quality of life: the capacity to experience and the ability to control pain and suffering.[8] But we know that alienation and isolation cause pain too. As care providers and policy analysts, should we not be reaching for more than legal or clinical definitions of pain and suffering? If the answer is yes, how should we redefine these terms? What should be our objectives for controlling them? How can we break the isolation in which so many elders live?

The Canadian Constitution states that Canadians have these fundamental freedoms: freedom of conscience and religion, of thought, belief, opinion, expression, and association. It states further that everyone has the right to "life, liberty and security." In the United States, similar expressions underscore every person's right to "life, liberty and the pursuit of happiness." There, case law has clarified and reinterpreted these rights. In Canada, the courts and daily practice will now begin to interpret these freshly stated constitutional freedoms in particular contexts. What are the implications of these freedoms for elders, those who provide services to them, and those who write policies which affect them? How can we better remember what these freedoms mean in the particulars of an elder's daily life, and so better implement their intent?

We must push at the boundaries of these words: freedom of association, conscience, privacy, security. They are more than legal terms. The merely legal interpretations of these words cannot be the goals of ethical, responsible people. Laws, after all, describe only the minimum standards that we set for people and their behaviour. Our goals for our elders, our agenda as service and care deliverers, as policy analysts, and as ethically concerned individuals must surely reach for more.

By broadening our definitions of these words, we suggest the beginning of a new agenda:

We mean by freedom the right of our elders to the least restrictive alternatives. We should encroach on the liberties of another only as a last resort – because there really is no other way, not because it is more convenient for us.

It may be easier for us to "manage" elderly persons if they are in restraints or under our guardianship, but our convenience cannot justify restricting their liberty. Protection is second to freedom in a democratic society.

We mean by privacy both freedom from sexual harassment and freedom to express one's sexuality. We have a responsibility to ensure that elders in our care are not touched against their will. We must remember that elderly women *have* been raped; rape is not a sexual act but a violent crime against a vulnerable person. We must also remember that the need to love and be touched and feel intimacy does not diminish with age. We should take these needs seriously by using our energies to find privacy for loving elders, even in our crowded institutions.

We mean by the right to security the right to feel safe at home and when walking to the market. Fear reduces quality of life; it erodes a sense of well-being. I think of an 80-year-old woman living in her double-bolted home, a citadel with shades drawn day and night; an 84-year-old watching TV all night and sleeping by day; a 70-year-old being raped by the superintendent of her housing project and having to walk daily past his door during the weeks of the police investigation. The quality of their lives are profoundly diminished – they are not free even though they live in their own homes.

We mean by freedom of belief that we not presume an elder's incompetency when his/her choices differ from ours. The right to informed consent means being given all the information needed to make a prudent decision: discussions about treatment options mean little if people are not informed about their diagnosis *and* prognosis. Consenting means being able to make a choice; choice is irrelevant if people believe that their benefits will be withdrawn or that they will stop receiving care if they do not choose what their doctors think best. Informed consent is of value only if people can choose what *they* feel is right for them. Freedom of belief has meaning only if people can apply their personal values to all the decisions of their lives.

We mean by freedom of conscience that elders have the right to feel confident that their values about death and life worth living are respected. The physician who takes an elder's refusal of treatment as prima facie evidence of incompetence has missed the point; freedom to choose means the right to choose differently, to be eccentric even, to make a mistake. We must recognize that elders' decisions about their lives flow out of their personal values, just as ours do. And decisions about letting nature take its course reflect elders' beliefs about death, life worth living, and responsibility to others.

We mean by freedom of association the right to be with those whom they love while they are dying, and to participate in creation while they are living. So we will abandon visiting rules which arbitrarily set limits on hours, numbers, and age to suit our schedules. We will push hard against the tendency to imagine that all elders are alike. In earlier years preferences for people, for associations, and for privacy vary with individuals, and we should assume that these variations continue throughout life. It is unfair and irresponsible to let elders in our care remain trapped in a room – or with wardmates – simply because they are bed-ridden or confined to a wheelchair.

Our first responsibility "is of course to keep the aging population in good physical and mental health as long as possible" and provide "adequate health care," as stated by the National Advisory Council on Aging.[9] If we really believe that, then our faulty attempts need reshaping and redefinition. More is asked of us: by our emerging awareness of the subtle aspects of caring for others, and by our understanding of what is at stake for both our community-in-the-present and our community-in-the-future.

Rights and freedoms mean little if people do not feel affirmed – respected – as unique and growing individuals. We readily recognize inhumanity and blatant disregard for persons. It is obvious that an individual who is fed while lying in his feces and urine is being inhumanely treated. We understand the disrespect demonstrated by a nursing home administrator who refers to resident couples as "dear little people" and who expects them to ask permission to occasionally share a marital bed. But we need also to keep in mind that these more subtle situations are also disrespectful of person and, often, inhumane:

> – the 80-year-old woman whose report of her rape in her kitchen is not believed by family or authorities because "she is so old";
>
> – the 82-year-old whose only recreational choice is Bingo, a game she abhorred in earlier years;
>
> – the family from Halifax who arrives at their dying father's Victoria bedside asking physicians to disregard his wish that only comfort care be given;
>
> – the 76-year-old woman who so fears her changed neighbourhood that she triple-bolts her door, stays up through the night, and sleeps only in the day.

We can do better.

Soelle and Cloyes remind us that "our capacity to praise creation hinges on our capacity to involve ourselves in creation. No genuine affirmation can arise apart from participation. Only through participation in creation can we affirm it, cherish it, praise it."[10] Every person seeks to participate in creation. Our specific charge is to promote the environment in which all can continue to do this and experience well-being to the fullest degree possible, despite age, circumstance, or disability. Our responsibility as ethical care providers is to create the environment in which our elders can continue to participate in creation as we ourselves do. This is our agenda.

NOTES

1 I am grateful to Ronald Philip Preston, who in *The Dilemma of Care: Social and Nursing Adaptations to the Deformed, the Disabled and the Aged* (New York: Elsevier 1979) has given us the parallel of Gregor to all alienated persons. My discussion here draws heavily from his work, in which he retells Kafka's story about Gregor (*The Metamorphosis*).
2 Ibid., 4–5
3 Ibid.
4 Ibid., 36
5 Ibid., 34
6 Dorothee Soelle and Shirley A. Cloyes, *To Work and to Love: Theology of Creation* (Philadelphia: Fortress Press 1984)
7 Julius Richmond, *Healthy People: The Surgeon General's Report on Health Promotion* (U.S. Department of Health, Education and Welfare 1979) 71
8 Law Reform Commission of Canada, *Sanctity of Life or Quality of Life* (Protection of Life Series Study Paper 1979) 70
9 National Advisory Council on Aging, from a Council discussion on schedule in preparation for the Canadian Report to the 1982 World Assembly on Aging, 7
10 Soelle and Cloyes, *To Work and to Love,* 1

3

Ethics and Aging: Trends and Problems in the Clinical Setting

DAVID ROY

Am I not wanted at all by anyone, anywhere? It is getting late.

AUTHOR UNKNOWN

Aging challenges the ethos, morality, and ethics of a community. *Ethos* comprises our governing perceptions, assumptions, and beliefs about the origin, destiny, and meaning of human life, and about the goals and means of the institutions we have fashioned to maintain community life. Ethos is a foundation of moral living. It partially determines a hierarchy of values. We often differ quite sharply about what is of greater or lesser importance in life, about which values may be sacrificed and which are to be maintained, perhaps at any cost. *Morality* is based upon our governing values, purposes, and goals.

Ethos and morality need *ethics*. Ethics works out the judgments that have to be made when moral design confronts constraints on the real possibilities available to individuals and societies. Ethics applies the norms shaped by fundamental perceptions and governing values to resolve value conflicts in a real world marked by limitations. These may affect the range of real possibilities open to people, as well as their personal and moral development.

Clinical ethics works on the resolution of value conflicts at the bedside; more generally, on the resolution of conflicts arising from uncertainty or conflicts between views on how best to care for those who are sick, weak, suffering, or facing death. The patient's biography – his or her clinical situation, relationships, life plans, beliefs, perceptions, persuasions, and total life interests – is the bottom line criterion of clinical ethics. Clinical ethics rejects using the patient as a battlefield for conflicting moral persuasions and traditions. Its aim is to achieve the most accurate description of the patient possible. Decisions or policies based on partial or false descriptions that do not match patients' real clinical interests and life plans court injustice. The maxim of clinical ethics is that each case contains its own resolution. Understand the patient as comprehensively as possible, and the balance of factors required to resolve an ethical uncertainty or dilemma will emerge.

This paper is more than an essay in clinical ethics. It must necessarily adopt a perspective broader than the bedside if the older person there is to be sensitively perceived and humanely treated.

HOW DO WE SEE THE AGED?

As a crabbit old woman? This was the key phrase in a poem left by an old lady after she died in the geriatric ward of Ashludie Hospital, near Dundee, Scotland. She addressed her poem to nurses, asking with the opening line what they saw when they looked at her. A crabbit old woman, withdrawn, passive, slovenly, and uncommunicative? She then asked them to open their eyes because, if that was what they saw, they were not looking at her. She proceeded to tell them who she was: still a small child, a young girl of sixteen, a bride, a mother, a lonely woman whose children had left home, a grieving woman whose husband had died. As an old woman, from whom grace and vigour had departed, she was still all of these persons she once had been. She vigorously assured them that in her old carcass a young girl still dwelt.[1]

How *do* we view the aged? Will we ever see in an old woman or an old man all of the persons they once were and still are? How can we, if we are blinded by what Robert N. Butler, MD, has called the myths of aging, unproductivity, disengagement, inflexibility, senility, and serenity?[2] These myths are perception filters through which pass, indeed, a great number of truths about the aged. What they filter out, however, is an older person's unique individuality. When we miss seeing that, we are close to discrimination and mind-crippling bias.

Bias, a reduction of affirmations and decisions to unexamined perceptions, is how we come to diverge systematically from the truth. Bias is the bane of scientific research and every effort is made, such as randomized and multiple blind clinical trials, to reduce its devastating effects on our search for reliable medical knowledge. Bias can also cause us to diverge systematically, and tragically, from that which is right and demanded by the primordial canons of humanity. This is the threat of the bias of "ageism."

> Ageism can be seen as a process of systematic stereotyping of and discrimination against people because they are old, just as racism

> and sexism accomplish this with skin color and gender. Old people are categorized as senile, rigid in thought and manner, old fashioned in morality and skills. . . . Ageism allows the younger generations to see older people as different from themselves; thus they subtly cease to identify with their elders as human beings.[3]

What efforts can we possibly make to limit the devastating effects of this kind of bias?

AGING: WHAT MAY WE EXPECT ON THE LARGE SCALE AND IN THE LONG RUN?

We need an accurate predictive framework to plan constructively and on time to meet the demands that the care of the aged will make upon us, and especially upon others who are younger than we are. These perspectives and goals are as much an ethical demand as is the sensitive perception of a unique individual in an old body.

It is very difficult to determine accurately what we should expect about aging on the large scale, and about the moral demands the care of the aging will make upon us and our communities in the long run. There are both controversies and some fairly certain trends.

One earlier model of the future curve of aging, that proposed by James F. Fries, emphasizes a very optimistic emergence of a pattern of natural death at the end of a natural life span. Geometrically, this model predicts that a squaring of the survival curve will be followed by a squaring of the curve of suffering and lingering inactive and dependent life. This "compression of morbidity" model means that the onset of infirmity will be increasingly delayed till the very end of life, indeed, of a long life. The Fries model suggests "a radically different view of the life span and of society, in which life is physically, emotionally, and intellectually vigorous until shortly before its close, when, like the marvelous one-hoss-shay, everything comes apart at once and repair is impossible."[4]

As one may suspect, this is all probably just a bit too good to be true. Models are as weak as their governing assumptions, and some of the assumptions of the Fries model have come under heavy critical fire.

There is no conclusive evidence that the human life span – the maximum survival potential of the human organism – is as genetically defined or limited as the replicative capacity of laboratory-cultured human cells. "Natural" death, that is, death in the absence of disease, seems to remain a hope rather than a frequent occurrence. Current trends indicate that life expectancy is on the rise and mortality rates are decreasing. The most rapid decline in mortality rates is to be found in the age group eighty-five years and older.[5] The number of persons in this age group of the "oldest old" could more than triple between 1980 and 2020.[6] The oldest old may take longer to die over the next forty years than the Fries model would lead one to expect.

If the oldest old increase dramatically in numbers over the next forty years, they will also be those who are most prone to chronic diseases. The postponement of first appearance of these disabling conditions in the elderly will not likely happen naturally. In the absence of major research advances in preventive, restorative, and palliative medicine, shrinkage of the period of suffering for the elderly – "compression of morbidity" – is not to be expected. Quite the contrary if the oldest old, as mentioned above, may be expected to take longer to die than the rectangularization of mortality curve hypothesis would predict.

This rapidly summarized critique of the assumptions underlying the Fries model suggests quite a different picture of the future of the aged. In view of current growth and mortality rates in the population of the aged and oldest old, we may have to expect "that the average period of diminished vigor will probably increase, that chronic diseases will probably occupy a larger proportion of our life span, and that the needs for medical care in later life are likely to increase substantially."[7] If medical needs increase, costs will rise. Who, if anyone, will be able to cover these costs? One study observes that: "The enormous costs of medical care cannot be borne by individuals living on limited post-retirement income and assets. Hence, the quantity and quality of life in extreme old age are broad-ranging social problems, with government being viewed more and more as the agent responsible for the financial needs of the aged."[8]

On what basis will we judge the ethics of using increasing portions of limited resources for the general and medical care of the aged and of the oldest old? Will the microethical imperative of sensitively recognizing a unique human individual in a crumbling body, and of behaving consistently with this recognition, come into conflict with the macroethical requirement of justice in maintaining the common good? We may well have to think more profoundly than ever before on what the common good will mean over the next forty years. Can the content of the common good change with time and with historical and social circumstances?

CARE OF THE AGED: WILL THEY BE WORTH THE COST?

Scarce resources and competing demands require that some measurable value be assigned to various programmes that save lives. A cost-benefit analysis uses money as the unit of measurement of value. One of the approaches of a cost-benefit analysis, the so-called human capital approach, assumes "that the value to society of an individual's life is measured by future production potential, usually calculated as the present discounted value of expected labor earnings.''[9] However, what discount rate will be used to convert future earnings into present values? The results of the choice of rate can be very interesting and have far-reaching ethical implications. Landefeld and Seskin have shown that the 1977 U.S. dollar value of males aged one to four is $405,802 if a discount rate of 2.5 per cent is used. This value sinks to $31,918 if a discount rate of 10 per cent is chosen.[10]

The monetary worth of economically non-productive and consumption-intensive elderly people drops dramatically when calculated in this way. Jerry Avorn has observed one result of the cost-benefit approach applied to calculate the ''worth'' of the elderly. In terms of 1977 U.S. dollars, ''a program that would save the life of an 85-year-old man (thus yielding a benefit of $943) compares poorly with one that would save a 32-year-old (yielding a benefit of $205,062).''[11] J. P. Acton has observed ''that society is made better off by the death of those whose expected net present value is negative.''[12] He has also emphasized that people are neither machines nor the chattel of the state or of an economy.

If the implications of this and similar lines of reasoning were adopted as morally normative, we could easily reach conclusions that are morally intolerable. Avorn has sketched one possible terminus of this way of thinking.

> The logic of the human-capital argument would thus be perfectly consistent with the concept that euthanasia (or at least nontreatment) after retirement is the geriatric intervention with the most favorable benefit-cost ratio. As Woody Allen has noted with equal insight, ''Death is a great way to cut down on expenses.'' Absent from this view are the notions of compassion, rights, one's debt to one's parents and forebears, or any sense of altruism or equity.[13]

A patient's clinical condition, not his or her individual age or age category, should be the governing criterion for decisions about which technologies, procedures, and services are appropriate. The claim that we often overmedicalize our care of the elderly can be amply documented. This claim, however, is not a basis, nor is it an excuse, for proposals to allocate resources according to the characteristic needs of different stages in the life cycle.

A danger lurks in the notion of concentrating rescue and life-extending technologies on the earlier stages of the human life cycle. Though most thoughtful persons would agree with the emerging ethical trend *against* mindless extension of life when the cerebral basis for consciousness and communication has been irreversibly destroyed, the tendency to equate elderliness with senility must be unmasked and checkmated. Proposals to identify life-extending technologies as most appropriate for the early or middle stages of life can easily collapse into discrimination against the elderly. These proposals are ethically not very promising or wise.

The challenge of caring for the oldest will soon force all of us, if we are not already so challenged, to come out with a moral clarification about what kind of a community or society we are. Will the oldest old find themselves refugees from an increasingly decivilized state and society? The oldest old have a unique vocation. Only they can enlighten us all about the meaning and the demands, the losses and the fulfillments of the full curve of human life's experience. Nurturing that vocation and assuring the economic, social, and cultural conditions for its flowering are essential for the advance of a society into civilization.

WHAT DOES DYING WITH DIGNITY MEAN WHEN YOU ARE OLD?

Blaise Pascal has said that a human being, even when subjected to the laws of nature that dictate descent into death, remains superior to the entire universe. This is so because a human being can know that he dies, while the universe knows nothing about what it does. Though the dignity of a human being does not consist in thought alone, how can one's dying be an expression of human and personal dignity if it has no chance to be the final expression of the meaning one has given to life and to love?

A model of *dying with dignity* would include at least the following elements:

– dying without a frantic technical fuss and bother to squeeze out a few more moments or hours of biological life, when the important thing is to live out one's last moments as fully, consciously, and courageously as possible;
– dying without that twisting, racking pain that totally ties up one's consciousness and leaves one free for nothing and for no one else;
– dying in surroundings that are worthy of a human being who is about to live what should be one's "finest hour." The environment of a dying patient should clearly say: the technical drama of medicine has receded to the background to give way to the central human drama, the drama, as the poet would say, of a unique human being "wrestling with his God";
– dying in the presence of people who know how to drop the professional role mask and relate to others simply and richly as a human being;
– dying with one's eyes open. No games, no pretense. We find and give to one another the courage to admit what is happening. A human being who can do this is already ahead of dying and superior to death;
– dying with one's mind open. The really hard questions that rattle the bedrock of our dreams and hopes face us unanswered at the time of dying. To

die firmly holding on to these questions, to refuse to latch on to some little myth designed to render these questions harmless and rob them of their power to echo through the soul, is what dying with an open mind demands; – dying with one's heart open. This I saw in a young woman dying of cancer. She gave us something of herself that reached beyond her death and that death could not take away. She made us want to live courageously and to live for others.

Reality is always too varied and complex to fit neatly into any one model of what dying with dignity means. The model may work well for a conscious and competent patient. But how do we respect the dignity of an unconscious or incompetent patient? What do we do when a fully conscious and reasonable patient refuses treatment that would definitely prolong life? What does respect for dignity demand or permit when patients are young and in deep, irreversible coma or are old and in deep, irreversible senility? Does dying with dignity mean that we do everything clinically possible to maintain an old person right down to the last centimetres of the Alzheimer curve of degeneration?

MAY WE ALLOW OR HELP THE OLD TO DIE?

''Dying with dignity'' has dominated the last ten years of medical practice, medical ethics, and medical law. It is often far from clear what that slogan should mean in hospitals that have become theatres for the deployment of a complex life-prolonging technology needing the services of many specialized persons. The sick and possibly dying person represents a cluster of clinical challenges woven into the pattern of a unique personal history. That history of desires, plans, achievements, loves, and hopes, not just health and biological survival, is thrown into question when devastating illness strikes and death threatens. That unique person, certainly weak and possibly frightened and confused, should be not only the object of the clinical decisions that have to be made but also the norm of the fundamental human choices that define the meaning of clinical activity at the extremes of life.

However, who is to make these choices and how are they to be made in a highly pluralistic society and in highly specialized hospitals? When should efforts to prolong or save a patient's life be stopped? On what moral basis should these decisions be made? How is the responsibility for such decisions to be shared? If it is morally justifiable to let a patient die, why is it not morally justifiable to hasten a patient's death?

The reappearance of groups promoting active euthanasia and ''rational'' suicide reveals levels of desperation that mark profound societal discord about important matters. The ways we deal with the dying, the terminally ill, and those whom medicine can save but not cure are in question. The controversy is about life, not just about ideas.

Dying with dignity has become a slogan of opposition to degrading and useless technological prolongations of biological life when a patient's organism, though still minimally functional, no longer supports or permits the exercise of intelligent and personal control over the events of his life. All would agree that it is an appalling degradation of human dignity to treat a person as a mere object. We readily accept this as a moral basis for our dealings with one another in other phases of life. The slogan "dying with dignity" is a call to respect this moral foundation in our relationship with those who are dying.

Biological existence in human beings is a condition for higher levels of development and achievement. Bernard Lonergan has expressed this point as follows: "Man develops biologically to develop psychically, and he develops psychically to develop intellectually and rationally. The higher integrations suffer the disadvantage of emerging later. They are the demands of finality upon us before they are realities in us."[14]

When an old person is in an irreversible state of advanced senility, we witness development in reverse. The "higher integrations" to which Lonergan refers are no longer possible. They have disappeared. These persons cannot think, reason, decide, choose, speak, communicate, or maintain interpersonal relationships. The question may be phrased sharply: if biological existence in these older persons cannot achieve its higher human purposes, need we make major medical efforts to maintain this biological existence? Need we give antibiotics to cure pneumonia in an irreversibly senile patient? Should we do this?

Morally justifiable acts in one kind of relationship may be immoral in another. The doctor-patient relationship obviously justifies high-risk invasions of the bodily integrity of human beings, acts that would be criminal outside this relationship. What acts do the medical mandate justify when a patient is deteriorating beyond medicine's ability to cure? Are there any moral limits to the measures a doctor may take to alleviate pain, suffering, and a lingering process of dying? A patient, conscious and lucid, may request rapid and painless death from a doctor. In certain extreme cases of cancer, with respect to certain unsalvageable infants, and when faced with certain irreversibly senile patients in a state of painful and prolonged dying, doctors themselves may ask whether waiting for death to occur defines the limit of their moral and professional duty.

Several years ago, Dr. J. Freeman asked: "In those rare instances where the decision has been made to avoid 'heroic' measures and to allow 'nature to take its course,' should society not allow physicians to alleviate the pain and suffering and help nature to take its course – quickly?''[15] Freeman's question concerned the care of neonates. The times when this question arises are not rare in the care of the old who are chronically ill and cerebrally degenerating.

How is such a question to be answered? By measuring the proportion of benefits to damages? In this event, whose benefits and damages enter into the ratio? Only the patients'? Do we need to take a broader view and seek to answer the question by considering long-term consequences of an act of ''mercy'' that amounts to killing patients who fail to die rapidly enough for their own good or, perhaps, for the good of others? Should a society give such power to medicine or to any profession? If we were to justify some acts of humanitarian infanticide or geronticide, are we also capable of establishing generally acceptable and non-arbitrary limits to the putative medical mandate to shorten ''useless dying curves'' by direct termination of life? Do we try this as an experiment and closely monitor the results? Do we, on the basis of a fear that ''things might get out of hand,'' decree that no one, doctors included, is ever morally justified in terminating a patient's life?

Some, perhaps many, would hold that such a decree is not arbitrary at all. It would simply be an expression of the most basic of all principles, namely that no human being has dominion over the life of another. However, the film *Breaker Morant* demonstrated the thesis that, in war, situations arise that fall outside all existing rules. Surely similar situations arise in medicine? Should we then recognize these situations as exceptions to the dominion argument, act accordingly, and avoid public discussion of acts that cannot be generalized and hence cannot be regulated by any rule or law?

CONCLUSION

Decisions in extreme situations appeal necessarily to our deepest principles and beliefs. Moreover, though we share a common humanity, persons are unique, often remarkably different in what they value most highly in life. As we strive to build a clinical ethics on the basis of our common humanity the danger to be avoided is the production of an establishment ethics that leaves little freedom for moral minorities. As we strive to build an ethics capable of respecting personal originality, the danger to be aware of is the seduction of a facile relativism that ignores the bonds and the possibilities of our shared humanity.

These bonds are the foundation for an ethics of aging. This includes more than needed reform of our individual and social behaviour towards the retired and the oldest old. Our view of the aged, and the place we accord them in our community, shapes the present and the future of children and youth. A rich network of contacts with older people gives depth to a young person's past and growing sense of personal identity. Without a deep past, the future may seem both shallow and insecure. the quotation that opened this paper, spoken by one who was old, echoes throughout late-twentieth-century adolescence.

NOTES

1 The text of this untitled poem was published in the *Beacon House News,* a magazine of the Northern Ireland Association for Mental Health.
2 Robert N. Butler, *Why Survive?: Being Old in America* (New York: Harper & Row 1975) 6–11
3 Ibid., 12, quoted in Robert N. Butler and Myna I. Lewis, *Aging and Mental Health: Positive Psychosocial Approaches* (St. Louis: C.V. Mosby 1973)
4 James F. Fries, "Aging, Natural Death, and the Compression of Morbidity," *New England Journal of Medicine* 303 (1980): 135
5 Edward L. Schneider and Jacob A. Brody, "Aging, Natural Death, and the Compression of Morbidity: Another View," *New England Journal of Medicine* 309 (1983): 854
6 Richard Suzman and Matilda White-Riley, "Introducing the 'Oldest Old'," *Milbank Memorial Fund Quarterly* 63 (1985): 179
7 Schneider and Brody, "Aging, Natural Death," 854
8 Ira Rosenwaike, "A Demographic Portrait of the Oldest Old," *Milbank Memorial Fund Quarterly* 63 (1985): 202
9 J. Steven Landefeld and Eugene P. Seskin, "The Economic Value of Life: Linking Theory to Practice," *American Journal of Public Health* 72 (1982): 556
10 Ibid.
11 Jerry Avorn, "Benefit and Cost Analysis in Geriatric Care," *New England Journal of Medicine* 310 (1984): 1297
12 Jean-Paul Acton, "Measuring the Monetary Value of Lifesaving Programs," *Law and Contemporary Problems* 40 (1976): 53, note 17
13 Avorn, "Benefit and Cost Analysis," 1297
14 Bernard J. Lonergan, *Insight: A Study of Understanding* (New York: Philosophical Library 1957), 625
15 John M. Freeman, "Is There a Right to Die – Quickly?" *Journal of Pediatrics* 80 (1972): 905

4

Ethical Aspects of Aging: Justice, Freedom, and Responsibility

JOHN C. BENNETT

I am no authority on the social science of gerontology but I have one advantage over most of those who are, because I am a specimen of the class of people they are studying.[1] I am an octogenarian and live in a retirement community in which I can observe the aging of my 300 neighbours as well as my own aging. I have taught and written about Christian ethics during most of career and I try to relate that teaching to my present situation.[2]

In the most general terms, I think that there are at least three ethical concerns that are applicable to the lives of those who are considered elderly. The first is that society as a whole should do justice to them. Some progress has been made in that regard. By justice I do not mean merely a fair application of existing rules, but a transforming justice that raises the level of dignity and opportunity of all who are neglected and deprived. The second concern is that they should have freedom, freedom to be themselves as far as this is possible, freedom from unnecessary dependencies, freedom from paternalism. I realize that those who live longest, or who become ill in body, or who, more sadly, lose mental awareness and memory become necessarily dependent and that there must be a benign paternalism. Sometimes these misfortunes are brought on or worsened by the subhuman conditions of life to which older people are often subjected. Geriatric medicine has shown that symptoms of senility can often be reversed by diet, by correcting a wrong mixture of medicines, and by better human relations. After one has made allowance for the special problems of the most advanced in age, there should be a great deal of emphasis on freedom for the elderly as a group. My third moral concern for them is that they live responsibly. I emphasize that they should have as much responsibility as possible for the conditions of their lives, a sense of responsibility for the welfare of the elderly as a group, and responsibility for their immediate community and for the decisions, often political, of the larger society.

Prior to all these moral concerns that touch the lives of the elderly is the need to overcome the stereotypes through which people so often see them and through which they so often see themselves. We need to begin by recognizing how wide the age span of the elderly has come to be. It begins at 65 and extends to any year you want to name between 65 and 100. I think that it is usually suggested that this long period be divided, so far as the limitations of age are concerned, into the years between 65 and 75 and the years from 75 and beyond. My own experience of living among many elderly people has led me to put the dividing line at about 80. Also, I am impressed by the liveliness and capacity to make contributions to society which many people retain long after they reach 80. In any case, we need in this context to avoid stereotypes that become self-fulfilling prophecies about the possibilities of elderly people during this wide span of years.

There comes a time in the lives of many when they should be helped to decide to move to a less independent kind of life. My own retirement community has learned from experience that it is often best for persons to do this while they have the strength to make the most of the possibilities that are open to them. Decisions for people from 85 to 95 are extremely difficult, as one wants to hang on to home and possessions and ways of life which have been valued so much over the years. Even here freedom of choice should not be lost before it becomes essential to give it up, for the health of the person involved and for the well-being of his or her neighbours. Often, those who hang on too long to their independence exploit the kindness of their neighbours.

There is a common stereotype about older people in general which regards them as unhealthy, ingrown, inactive, out of date in their ideas, rigid, and vulnerable to senility. These ideas are often the cause of great injustice to persons whom they do not fit, injustice in the social provisions made for them. This is especially true if they have had a temporary experience of serious illness or of some kind of disorientation. Being on guard against such injustice is very important in the case of institutions for the elderly. The way people are treated often takes away their own sense of self-worth, and there is a vicious circle as this inner loss causes the treatment by others to be more dehumanizing.

Justice, freedom, and responsibility are closely interrelated. Without justice in the form of considerable economic security for the elderly, both freedom and the capacity to assume responsibility are greatly limited. The enormous increase in the proportion of people over sixty-five, most of whom are economically non-producers, has raised acute questions concerning what society as a whole should do to provide such economic security. In an earlier period, it could be expected that most elderly parents would either live with their children or in other ways be supported by them. This is now much less frequently the case. The children less often live in large houses in the same communities where their parents have lived and have friends and other relatives. For three generations to live together in small houses and apartments can be very difficult for all of them, especially when they are in cities strange to the grandparents. One cannot generalize about what the best arrangements for parents are. It is often fortunate when they live independently but near one or more children. During a late period of crippling illness, it may be best for them to live with their children when this is possible. But this may also be either impossible or unwise.

One solution is the kind of retirement community in which I live, where most people live independently, where there are two levels of care available, one involving nursing care and the other merely some helps for living and twenty-four hour monitoring. Such a community offers the advantage of bringing together people who face many of the same problems, with opportunities for a great deal of mutual help, understanding, and companionship. One drawback is that the segregation of older people leads to too great a segregation of generations. The location of the retirement community is an important factor.

It is very difficult for children to decide that their parents should live in a nursing home because these homes have such a bad reputation for dehumanizing treatment and warehousing of people. But good ones can be found and this may be the best solution for those who are totally or almost totally dependent. Children have a great responsibility to help choose the nursing home and to be advocates for their parents. When elderly people in that situation have no family near them, churches and other groups or institutions need to assume the role of advocates. Ideally, we should provide considerable independence for the elderly as long as this is physically and mentally possible, but this should not mean that their children do not continue to have an important role. Their love and acts of caring, their presence, either frequently or at special times of illness or other emergencies, are of great importance for parents, for their morale and for help in meeting life's problems.

What I have just said presupposes that elderly people should have as much economic independence as possible. Justice and compassion call for this from society. The elderly have made their contribution to society and after retirement they deserve to have the means of livelihood and the kind of consideration that I have emphasized. They also need medical care more than younger people, and provisions for this are an important part of economic security. In the United States, the Social Security system has been the largest and most reliable federal movement toward social justice. President Reagan at one time talked about making Social Security voluntary, but as a politician, he put such ideas aside. The most that can be done by politicians to reduce Social Security benefits would be to reduce the rate of increase in relation to inflation, and this has been done. Social Security by itself does not usually provide complete economic independence, but it is an enormous help for the majority. However, there are millions of poor women who never made enough to have much income from Social Security. This is one reason why in the United States we often speak of the feminization of poverty.

Medicare is a more recent breakthrough which, after a deductible that grows too fast, takes over most of the burden of hospital costs for many weeks. It pays a fixed amount to doctors but they generally bill patients for considerably more than that amount – an unsolved problem in the States which government has gone far to solve in Canada. Medicare is available to elderly people regardless of their means. It must be distinguished from Medicaid, which is available to those whose income level makes them eligible for what we call "welfare," regardless of age. Budget stringencies often reduce the quality of care. Even under Medicare, we may have our freedom to choose doctors and hospitals seriously reduced. The great deficiency in the case of Medicare is that it makes no provision for long-term custodial care that often is required for many years. Many people with middle incomes spend most of what they have in the first year or two and are forced to go on Medicaid. Children often accept it as the only way of providing for a parent's long illness.

I have used illustrations from the United States to indicate how one individualistic country has moved to provide much more economic independence for the elderly than they had in earlier periods. The idea of a national system of medical insurance used to be talked of, but today we seldom hear of it because of the exorbitant costs of medicine today and the federal budgets deficits. The last time I remember hearing about such a system was when Senator Edward Kennedy used the Canadian system as a model. My hope is that Canada will continue to be a national laboratory in which schemes of medical care for the whole population can be tested, and that the United States may learn from those experiences.

When this subject of economic independence for the elderly is discussed, we are reminded of the decreasing number of producers who must bear the burden of supporting an increasing number of economic non-producers. This problem is exacerbated by the immense defence budget in the United States, and I hope that reductions in that budget will make more resources available for people of all ages. There are two things that the economically productive generations should bear in mind. One is that those who feel responsibility for the welfare of their parents will be greatly helped in the discharge of that responsibility by such programs as the Social Security system and Medicare, which have their equivalents in all industrialized democracies. Also, those who support such systems for the elderly while they are engaged in economic production are creating or preserving institutions from which they will benefit when they become older, and one can expect that they will live longer than the generation that now receives such benefits.

Much can be said about the relation between the freedom of elderly people to be themselves and to be true to their own convictions and a degree of self-restraint that is desirable when they confront quite different ideas of conduct among their children and grandchildren. I doubt if there has been a time in which mores and ideas about what is morally acceptable in personal life have changed so rapidly. There are many shifts in priorities, if not in basic values, and these call for a great deal of understanding from those of us who are older. The younger generation is not always right. The latest style of life is not always the best. I am not suggesting that older people give in to the kind of moral relativism that suggests that anything goes. And yet there is often need of mutual tolerance. Common sense, consideration for the freedom of others, recognition that there are societal changes that account for some differences in personal behaviour between generations, living with honest differences of opinion – these are all needed. How they are to be reconciled with the freedom of those of us who are older to be true to our own convictions and scale of values is something that calls for playing by ear, for tact and understanding.

There is one important public issue that comes up when we think of freedom of choice, especially among the younger members of the older population. This is the issue of retirement. There is such a difference among jobs that one cannot generalize too much. Many jobs call for heavy work and are so physically taxing that either early retirement from them or a change of work is essential for the health of the worker. Actually, in the United States retirement before the age of sixty-five is often desired. This is often true concerning jobs that are especially dull. Yet when retirement comes, it often becomes another form of dullness. People have nowhere to go in the morning. Associations on the job are missed. In the case of jobs that provide opportunities for creative ability or that are very interesting (which would be true of many kinds of professional jobs), retirement may be a serious deprivation. I do not know what it is like to have a job that gives one great power and then be suddenly deprived of it at sixty-five and given enormous deferred payments of pensions and other fringe benefits as bribes for accepting retirement. I have often thought that seldom has a class of powerful people yielded power in exchange for comfort while they still have a full capacity to work, as leaders of business do today. They are a generation away from the great founding entrepreneurs who often stayed on the job until death. One of the best solutions in some cases, and this would be true of academic jobs, which

I know best, may be to move to part-time work. This enables one to retain associations and to do fresh work even though compensation may be limited since one is already drawing a pension. In this way, one might step down from a position of power in an institution and continue some teaching and research. Such a programme preserves the contributions of able people and enables them to have both a community and the stimulus for creative work, while it opens the door for the advancement of younger scholars.

Twenty-five years ago, the idea of disengagement[3] seemed to many to be the ruling idea in gerontology, but now its inadequacies are clear even to some of its original advocates. True, there must be disengagement in some respects, and the need for this increases as one's capacity for action decreases and as one outlives more and more contemporaries. Also, one should not stay too close to one's former job if it involved much institutional decisionmaking, for to do so may embarrass one's successors. When I retired from Union Theological Seminary, I moved three thousand miles away to avoid being a problem to the institution. Not everyone need move so far! But after one has said what needs to be said about disengagement, two other things should be added. Some continuing engagement, even in another place, may still be desirable in order to retain one's identity and the unity of one's life, past and present. More important, there should be re-engagement. Retirement should not be one long vacation involving no new engagement with communities and institutions, with voluntary roles in new situations. Life should involve more leisure and, living in my retirement community, I envy my friends who have the greatest variety of interesting and often creative hobbies. I still spend my time doing much the same things that I did before I retired, writing and lecturing, and when I outgrow them I shall be at a disadvantage.

There are two areas of responsibility to which elderly people should be called as long as they have enough physical and mental strength. One of them is to do what they can to improve the conditions under which elderly people live. In one sense the elderly are a class because they have common interests and disabilities, and collective action, often political action, is necessary to improve their status and opportunities and provide access to remedies for their disabilities. In another sense they are not a class because all those of other generations who survive will become elderly and join that group. This means that when I work politically for the well-being of those who are now elderly, I am not seeking any exclusive gains for them but rather gains that will also be available to their successors, who will come from all social groups. Those who work for the welfare of the elderly, for economic justice and health for them, and for the improvement of institutions such as nursing homes, where many of them will end their lives, are working for the good of many millions now and for the welfare of others in the future. The elderly should avoid some actions that are contrary to the welfare of younger people, such as voting against bonds needed for schools. I am also shocked when they use their clout to keep children out of large residential areas through pressure on landlords or through covenants in the sale of property that exclude children from housing. To me this is a real sign of decadence. Local legislation is often sought to prevent such exclusive arrangements, and I hope that many of my generation will support it. Courts may be able to insist on equal protection for children.

Older people should not limit themselves in their public activity to the issues that especially affect their welfare. A great many of them have a freedom that they did not have during their years of employment to act on the basis of new thinking about the institutions and policies of their society, local, regional, and national as well as cultural and political. Employed people, even in a free society, are often very limited when it comes to going against the stream on political issues. Security in their jobs, possible promotion, and the avoidance of objectionable pressure from colleagues and superiors may depend on following the company line on controversial issues. People at the top often have more freedom than people in the bureaucratic middle or anyone who hopes to be on the way up. It may be different in Canada, but in the United States there are millions of people, many of them economically privileged, who really do not have free speech or the opportunity for free associations in connection with controversial public issues. Often they do not realize this, as their minds are formed from early days by pressures to which they become unconscious. When one is retired and on pension, with no firing or promotion in the picture, one has freedom to take fresh looks at the conventional wisdom in one's circle. Sometimes the issues that affect the economic security of older citizens will trigger a fresh look at choices in general.

What could be more fitting than for those who have lived most of their life spans to do all they can to save future generations from nuclear war? They would have many allies among younger people. At the moment, it seems that there we have a better chance than ever before to change the thinking in the United States as a whole. I am sure that Canada would be ahead on this issue because anti-Sovietism and the military defence of the west has not been so much a part of its political life. Two new developments are favourable: the pioneering and courageous witness of the Catholic bishops and the increasing awareness of the indirect and long-term consequences of nuclear war, such as the effect upon the earthly and atmospheric environment. I need not go into this, but we have here an open situation which may make possible a real change in attitudes and new policies in North America.[4] Older people, with their greater freedom to speak and to act, have an area of important action prepared for them.

There are innumerable opportunities for older people to learn more about public issues through programs of continuing education. The extraordinary success of Elderhostels shows what is possible in terms of formal opportunities for study and discussion of issues. Perhaps some of these, more than is the case today, should emphasize preparation to deal competently with the fateful political issues of justice and peace.

Older people will sometimes make use of political channels but they may more often act through their churches and through many voluntary organizations. The younger and stronger among them can do much more for those who are weaker and more dependent. In my retirement community I see this taking place daily in many ways that are beautiful and self-giving. Those who need help receive it, and those who give help gain meaning in their lives. Neighbours do help neighbours. The ultimate example of this kind of helping is seen when one spouse helps another to live in weakness and in sickness. The responsibility of older people ranges from political work to prevent nuclear war to the helping of a weaker person by a stronger one.

An idea common in high government circles in the United States may be suggested by what I have just said, but seems to me to be quite wrong: a general preference for voluntary as opposed to legally supported public provisions to meet the large-scale needs of older persons. This emphasis on voluntarism as the main method of meeting such needs has a fine moral sound. Is it not a better sign of personal generosity for people to give to the needy, young, or old voluntarily rather than for them to be taxed in order to provide people with access to medical care or to provide children with lunches as a matter of justice? It seems to me a serious error to answer "yes" to that question. Such voluntary aid cannot be expected to be enough to meet the needs of deprived and neglected people. But more serious is the capriciousness of such voluntary aid. It is unjust when large groups of people, except in emergencies, must depend for health and the necessities of life on the unstable and passing impulses of generosity of private persons rather than upon the sense of justice of the community to which they belong. Laws cannot take the place of personal virtues, but one personal virtue is willing to be taxed for the sake of the common good.

I shall conclude by discussing two issues that are the most difficult of all, issues about which there is not the beginning of consensus even among thoughtful and caring people. The first concerns the allocation of scarce medical resources, which are most often needed by that part of the population over sixty-five. The word triage has become important in our ethical vocabulary. It is a word that has its clearest meaning in simple situations such as disasters or emergencies when choosing from an overwhelming number needing medical treatment is an obvious problem, because the supply of medicine and the time of doctors are limited, and because there are both varying degrees of need and varying degrees of hope for success. A famine creates the need for such a choice. Now the extraordinary development of new therapies such as organ transplants makes this an almost everyday problem.

The second issue concerns the extent to which persons facing terminal illness and death, facing the possibility that their bodies may survive their minds for years, have a responsibility to prepare for the hastening of death under some circumstances.

I am indebted to a volume entitled *Triage and Justice*[5] by Gerald R. Winslow for a sensitive analysis of the various positions taken by thoughtful people on the allocation of scarce resources. Winslow mentions several principles which he calls "utilitarian": the principle of medical success; the principle of immediate usefulness, as in the case of doctors who can save other lives; the principle of conservation, concerning how much of the resources are needed in particular cases; the principle involving the responsibility of parents for children; and the principle of the general social value of the persons who might be chosen. He is most doubtful about the last, because of the very subjective nature of judgments about social value. He adds to these utilitarian principles suggestions about methods of choice that are based on the fundamental principle of the equal dignity of all persons. One of these is giving preference to those who arrive first, what he calls "queuing." Another is random selection. Lots can be drawn with priority given according to chance. The two approaches may come together if it is decided that random selection may be made among people who meet some objective test, such as the degree of need or chance for success, provided the situation makes such determinations possible. This analysis of various positions shows how difficult the problem of choice is.

How is all of this related to older people? For one thing, it is they who are very likely to be in greatest need. Chances of success are related to a person's basic health, which may be poorer among those of advanced age. This consideration often converges with another that has not been mentioned: life expectancy following therapy. I am here only raising a question and not trying to give an answer. When medical resources are scarce and financial resources limited, should the expected length of life be considered? I think that beyond some point in the upper age bracket, far above sixty-five, it is obvious that this should be considered, but where do we draw the line and who is to decide? Probably some committee representing the medical profession and the public should be involved, but what guidelines should it follow? Should I, in my eighties, encourage the judgment that my expected length of life after some forms of therapy would probably be too short and that the resources should be made available to persons who are younger? I am quite open to such a judgment and think that it would be responsible for me to throw my weight in that direction.

We are at the beginning of a long road that has many forks, and choices at each fork may increase in difficulty. The unbelievably rapid increase in medical knowledge and technology will confront us with new choices continually. Resources for some therapies will become less scarce, especially if artificial organs become available and capable of working successfully.

The story of the use of hemodialysis involving artificial kidneys is very instructive. Professor Winslow[6] reports that when this began in Seattle about 1960, only one in fifty of those who needed this treatment could be served. The local committee had to select according to criteria of its own and was deeply involved in the dilemmas of triage. In 1973 the federal government began to subsidize this therapy and it became widely available, almost a matter of routine for many still active persons. Winslow comments that the money spent on this procedure meant that there was less for other diseases, so that there was a kind of triage involving diseases to be emphasized, and this could be quite arbitrary!

Complicated and expensive therapies that become absorbed into ordinary life in this way will doubtless become more and more common. There will be limits because of costs to society. Do persons have the right to scarce resources for long-continued expensive treatment if they are able to pay for them? Should economic privilege entitle one to the use of scarce resources? There is no doubt that it does now, and I believe society should deliberately seek to move away from this. This will not be easy in countries where economic privilege gives medical advantages to people in ordinary situations, quite apart from crises.

My last issue is probably the most controversial. Do older people in their closing years have any responsibility for their death? Our traditions – religious, medical, and legal – would answer "no." I believe that the answer should be a qualified "yes." Most of the time we have no choice except that of taking good care of our health both in medical terms and, probably more important, in terms of our life-style. I can speak for people who have every reason to assume that they are living in their last decade, and for us the fear of death, or even concern about death, is very much overshadowed by fear that our bodies may survive our minds. It is overshadowed by the fear that we may have debilitating and dehumanizing forms of illness that may last for years and make life only a burden for us if we remain conscious, and a very difficult burden for those close to us whether or not we are conscious. The miracles of medical science make it possible for our bodies to live very long and there are situations in which death is a friend. We all know that this is true.

I should add that a long and even painful terminal illness does not necessarily have these characteristics. It may be a time of inner growth and even of victory, and it may lead to deeper and richer relations with others. It may give others life and hope.

The latest approach to a new consensus about what should be done in the case of long, hopeless, and painful bodily survival without mental awareness and meaningful relations with others is that artificial life supports be discontinued. Adjectives about the means used, extraordinary or heroic, may become dated as the extraordinary becomes ordinary with the progress of medical science. At the Massachusetts General Hospital, according to Professor William May,[7] patients are divided into four groups and the fourth group is treated as follows: "all therapy can be discontinued though maximum comfort to the patient may be continued or instituted." Extraordinary and ordinary methods of treatment are discontinued when it is believed that it is in the best interests of the patient to be allowed to die. It may be a step beyond this to discontinue feeding. That is still a serious legal issue in some situations.

On the general question of discontinuing artificial life supports in some situations, Roman Catholic teaching has been helpful. Catholic moral theology has given much more attention to precise issues in medical ethics than has Protestant teaching about ethics. The general trend of Catholic teaching has been to preserve life at almost all costs, both at the beginning and end of a person's life. So this case of Catholic teaching, which goes back at least to Pope Pius XII, is helpful for all of us.

It seems to me that it is a highly responsible act for persons in the last years of life, or before, to leave instructions for family and doctors that they do not want to be kept alive by extreme artificial means beyond the period of life that is meaningful by any test. I know that "meaningful" is a slippery word, but surely there is a stage of bodily existence for which the word "meaningless" is a clear idea. The so-called "living will" is much used in the United States to give such a directive to family and doctors. It has no legal force but it can still give guidance to those who are willing to receive it. In several states, recent legislation gives some support to a living will which is signed periodically and fulfills certain conditions.[8]

When we move from this kind of passive euthanasia to direct action to hasten death, we have no guidance at all, and both the law and the medical profession are adamantly against it. I think that there will come new openness even to this as a religious and moral issue. But I can understand that for the law or for institutional practice in hospitals or nursing homes any systematic permissiveness will be extremely difficult. Careful Christian thinkers have begun to open the door to new thoughts about this. Paul Ramsey, who has always been very conservative about any departure from tradition on matters of life and death speaks in his book *The Patient as Person*[9] of two situations that may call for positive euthanasia: "cases of patients in deep and irreversible coma who can be and are maintained alive for many, many years," and "a kind of prolonged dying in which it is medically impossible to keep severe pain at bay." A thinker who makes more room for positive euthanasia is Daniel Maguire, in his book *Death by Choice*.[10]

Positive euthanasia or assisted suicide in cases of hopeless and long terminal illness would have the justification that it would be based upon consent. It is of the utmost importance that we distinguish between such terminal suicide and the suicide of temporary despair that is so common among young people. There are at times almost epidemics of the latter. I once heard Artur Rubinstein say on TV that when he was twenty-two he tried to commit suicide, but when he was in his nineties he thought that he was the happiest man in the world. Whatever one says on this subject, it should never be said in a way that might encourage that kind of suicide.

The churches have had a cruel record in dealing with suicide. It has been treated as one of the gravest sins against God.[11] Those who see suicide as assuming a prerogative that belongs to God, and thus being a grievous sin regardless of the situation, fail to realize that medical science, in its prolonging of life beyond the point where its human quality justifies efforts to preserve it, is itself a case of a human agency assuming a divine prerogative. Can we not see God as active both in medical science and in the human caring that seeks to counteract some of the results of the medical prolongation of life? The churches need to have new thoughts on this subject. Meanwhile, to their credit, they now usually deal with cases of suicide pastorally rather than judgmentally.

I believe that as a matter of personal conscientious choice, suicide may be a person's final act of responsible freedom. But problems arise when we think of it as a matter of policy for the state or for institutions that care for the elderly sick. We do not want to create a system that encourages it for utilitarian purposes or even suggests to the inconvenient sick that it is a duty! There is no general solution to this problem in sight, and all that is possible is tolerance for the personal conscience and renunciation by both church and society of the cruel judgmental attitude which has been so harmful to the families of suicides. The next generation will have to find new approaches to public policy on this final issue of personal freedom of choice.

NOTES

1 This paper is an independent one, but in 1981 I published a chapter entitled "Ethical Aspects of Aging in America" in a volume edited by William M. Clements: *Ministry with the Aging* (San Francisco: Harper & Row). Since I discussed some of the same themes, there is an inevitable overlapping of ideas, but this paper deals with them more fully.

2 The book that first gave me a helpful overall view of gerontology is by R.N. Butler, *Why Survive?: Being Old in America* (New York: Harper & Row 1975).

3 For "disengagement" see R.C. Atchley, *The Social Forces in Later Life* 2nd ed. (Belmont, CA: Wadsworth Publishing Company 1977) 209–11.

4 I have developed this idea that there are new hopes of changing attitudes about the use of nuclear weapons in "Nuclear Deterrence Is Itself Vulnerable," *Christianity and Crisis,* 13 August 1984, 296–301.

5 University of California Press 1982

6 Ibid., 16

7 D.H. Smith "The Right to Die and the Obligation to Care," in *No Rush to Judgement* (University of Indiana Press 1979)

8 A law passed in California (California Civil Code Sections 2410–42) provides a document entitled "Durable Power of Attorney for Health Care." A person initials one of three paragraphs which give in general terms that person's guidance to a named agent or alternates. He or she may write a paragraph. This power of attorney exists for seven years unless the person involved chooses a shorter period.

9 Yale University Press 1970, 161–64. Ramsey makes these statements, which for him are surprising, but in what follows he still seems to be making up his mind. He is sure about a long-continued comatose condition but adds a note in which he raises the question whether it is not possible always to suppress pain though often at the expense of the strength of the patient. Later he raises the question whether accepting these exceptions may weaken the medical profession's "impulse to save," and he concludes that it would not be the case.

10 Schocken Books 1974

11 Thomas Aquinas in *Summa Theologica* II, ii 64 5, 3 after a succession of arguments against suicide says that "It is perilous because it leaves no time for repentance." Given the presuppositions, that seems to clinch the matter. I was sent to that passage by J. Fletcher, *Morals and Medicine* (Princeton University Press 1954) 179.

NOTE: Attention should be given to Daniel Callahan, *Setting Limits: Medical Goals in an Aging Society* (Simon and Schuster 1987). This provocative book will have great influence on discussion of issues presented in this paper.

5

Paradigms of Aging: Growth versus Decline

JAMES E. BIRREN AND CANDACE A. STACEY

INTRODUCTION

The purpose of this paper is to review concepts of normal aging, including something of the biological, cognitive, and personality processes, leading to a discussion of individuals' potential for strategic adaptation or transcendence of limitations. We discuss the dynamics of the aging individual, who is characterized by both increments and decrements in capacities, and identify some of the parallel changes that may take place, such as the competence that may increase in late life while physical mobility may decline. Such differences in the direction of behavioural change may result in conflicts between subjective and objective models of aging, and may influence the value ascribed to older adults in our society.

This paper addresses two major questions: What does current scientific theory have to say about our objective and subjective models of aging? How are our models of aging relevant to ethical values of society? The point is made that models of aging must take into account the parallelism and inconsistencies in late-life development in order to present a comprehensive view of the older adult. Our explicit or implicit models of aging influence the roles made available to older adults in our society and the social supports to which the elderly have access.

BIOSCIENCE

This paper emphasizes the behavioural aspects of aging rather than the purely biological because it is in the behavioural domain that the valued characteristics of aging human beings come into focus. Ultimately, what matters is not whether our heart and bones are strong, but whether we derive a sense of meaning from a long life and are competent to deal with a changing environment that challenges us. Good health is a necessary element in a good life, but it by no means ensures one. In this sense, our characteristics are hierarchically arranged with biological health being a necessary but not sufficient condition for a meaningful, content, and competent life.

Almost all bioscientific models of aging take the view that aging is a deteriorative or decremental process (or set of processes) that brings organisms closer to death. Comfort (1956) linked the concept of aging to that of senescence, which he defined as "a change in the behavior of the organism with age, which leads to a decreased power of survival and adjustment" (p 190). An even narrower definition of aging was given by Handler (1960): "Aging is the deterioration of a mature organism resulting from time dependent, essentially irreversible changes intrinsic to all members of a species, such that with the passage of time, they become increasingly unable to cope with the stresses of the environment, thereby increasing the probability of death" (p 200). Explicitly or implicitly, in bioscientific models of aging one confronts the idea that aging organisms lose vitality and the capacity for self-repair, and are thereby less likely to survive. If the probability of dying did not increase with age or if it varied irregularly with age, there would be little reason to do research that attempts to identify underlying processes. It is important to distinguish between the increased probability of dying with age, particularly during terminal decline, and aging itself.

It is in the phase of terminal decline that such vital bodily functions as cardiac output, respiration, body temperature, and others may fall to such levels that the organism is not able to sustain behavioural and social functioning. Ill persons retreat from the world and, in extreme states, some of the terminally ill may lose the ability to reason and to recall memories which give individual character to lives. Terminal decline should be viewed as a phase of biological, psychological, and social decompensation and not as "normal aging." Prior to reaching critical terminal levels, there is a relatively independent level of functioning in which, for example, the oxygen-carrying capacity of the blood, the volume of blood discharged by the heart at each beat, and the amounts of oxygen and glucose that reach the brain do not really determine or limit the competence of the individual in adapting to environmental demands or engaging in behaviour appropriate to the social roles expected by community and family.

What has just been said is in keeping with observations made in a mental health study of normally aging men. In the normally healthy there is a great deal of autonomy of function in which biological factors are present as necessary conditions for human life but do not provide sufficient conditions for that which we would regard as the essence of human life. It is largely in the terminal stages of life that biological deterioration becomes the limiting or determining condition for other spheres of psychological and social functioning. It is in this phase of life that the biological definitions of aging by Handler (1960) and Comfort (1956) appear most appropriate, and in this stage of decompensation that a bioscientific model of aging seems most useful. This phase appears to be qualitatively different from that which went before in that a smaller number of critical biological variables determines the likelihood of survival and the entire sphere of the individual's functioning.

One view of aging in the biological sciences, more common in the 1950s than recently, is the idea that aging, analogous to radiation damage, represents the accumulation of the effects of random hits, until the cells and organism can no longer function. In this view, much of what happens to the individual over a life is adventitious, and we may age, to some degree, like an automobile whose useful life is terminated because of the accumulated dents, bangs, and wear and tear. We hear less often these days of error theories of aging even though the organism must still show the signs of random wear and tear. Perhaps this is the case because scientists have come to believe there is a more definitive pattern to the changes of age. Lansing (1959) quoted Robertson to the effect that natural death is always to some extent an accident but it occurs in organisms that are vulnerable to the event. So it is in discourse about the biology of aging that references are made to chance and accident as well as to the more deterministic forces of genetics. To the blend of genetic forces and accidents must also be added the patterning of behaviour with age due to culture, the DNA of society.

The significance of what has been said lies in the implication that the normally adapting, aging person will be expected to show wide ranges of autonomy in function over the adult years, in which, like a bottle of good wine, some qualities may be improving. However, one should not expect the process to continue indefinitely since the organism is, after all, a biological system. In a wine the qualities of taste, aroma, and colour need not change in synchrony. This discussion has introduced the thought that we should expect that in normally aging persons, social, psychological, and biological processes will show rather separate patterns until the phase of decompensation or terminal decline brings with it "non-negotiable" limits. By now enough caution has been introduced that we may expect to find some areas in which patterns of change with age are decremental, some areas in which they are incremental, and others in which characteristics remain unchanged with age over long periods. To proceed further in this discussion, we will examine some of the evidence from the behavioural sciences.

INTELLECTUAL CHANGE: INCREMENT OR DECLINE?

Research on intellectual change beyond the sixties generally reveals decline (Botwinick 1977). Cross-sectional studies comparing young and old subjects on the Wechsler Adult Intelligence Scale show a significant drop in the latter years on tasks which involve speed of response or nonverbal, perceptual-manipulative components. In contrast, performance of those tasks which rely heavily on verbal ability or general knowledge remain relatively stable into old age, or perhaps improve.

An extensive longitudinal investigation of intellectual change was begun in 1956 by Schaie (1980). This research involved the study of individuals in seven-year age groups from the twenties to the eighties over seven-year intervals. A major finding was that age differences observed in longitudinal research are smaller than those reported in cross-sectional research. There is, however, some evidence of a pattern of intellectual loss. In this study, reliable decrements on "word fluency," the most speeded task, first appeared at age 53, whereas no decrements were reported on verbal meaning between the ages of 74 and 81. Thus, decrements began to appear at an earlier age than found in previous research. Again, the pattern of loss was found to be consistent.

The general slowing observed in the behaviour of older adults becomes more apparent with increased task complexity. Older adults appear to take longer in decision making and in the monitoring of their performance. Birren et al. (1980) have suggested that slowing will ultimately be understood in terms of a single neurobiological process that affects all behaviour mediated by the central nervous system although expressed to different degrees in perception, reasoning, or motor performance. Of additional interest is the finding that older adults tend to do better on tasks that have some direct life relevance (Gardner & Monge 1977). Also, modest intellectual decline has been related to cardiovascular disease, low socioeconomic status, inactivity, and lack of intellectual stimulation (Schaie 1980). Finally, there is some indication that significant drops in intellectual ability are related to closeness to death, the influence of terminal decline.

The topics of learning and memory in old age have received considerable attention. The information-processing model has been particularly helpful in guiding research on age-related change. Memory research has generally reported minimal age differences in iconic, primary, and tertiary memory, unless reorganization or divided attention is necessary. Substantial age differences, however, have been found in the acquisition and retrieval of new information from secondary or long-term memory. Although there is some indication that memory function is related to the integrity of the biological system, this alone cannot account for the memory deficits observed in healthy, community-living elderly. Instead, deficits in the speed of processing, encoding, and retrieval have been implicated in the decreased memory performance of older adults (Salthouse 1980). Evidence for a retrieval deficit can be found in the consistent finding that age differences in recognition are much smaller than those for recall, implying that the information is stored but cannot be accessed. The ability to access stored information is enhanced considerably when retrieval cues are provided. Also, pacing the response phase of a task results in greater age differences, providing additional evidence for an age deficit in search and retrieval. Age differences are apparent, however, even under self-paced conditions. Ultimately, the processes of encoding and retrieval cannot be separated, since retrieval is largely dependent on efficient encoding. There is considerable evidence for age decrements in the use of encoding and organizational strategies.

In general, research involving ecologically valid tasks tends to show smaller age differences than research with laboratory tasks. Also to be considered are those contextual aspects, such as motivation and task familiarity, which play an important role in learning and memory.

Clearly, performance in memory, learning, attention, information-processing rate, and so on bear directly upon the older individual's problem-solving ability. As yet, we know little about how these processes work together in cognitive activities. As Rabbitt (1977) points out, a major difficulty in comparing and understanding the problem-solving literature is the absence of a "satisfactory taxonomy in which to discuss similarities or differences between rules, organizational procedures, etc., when these are operationally defined across different kinds of experiments" (p 613). There are age differences in problem solving which tend to increase with task complexity. Older adults are relatively poor at cognitive organization; however, they can significantly improve their performance with training, which suggests some degree of plasticity in cognitive functioning. Older adults appear to prefer simpler strategies, but there is little evidence that existing strategies are rigidly adhered to or inhibit the use of more sophisticated strategies (Rabbitt 1977). A number of studies have reported that older adults are more cautious than young ones (see, for example, Botwinick 1966). Rabbitt (1977) suggests that apparent cautiousness may reflect a difficulty in working appropriate solutions.

Other factors which influence problem-solving performance include age-related deficits in the rate of information processing and perceptual organization. Older adults tend to require more time to scan and evaluate visually complex displays (Rabbitt 1968). This increased time interacts with memory. The greater the length of time spent in scanning, the greater the probability that important information stored in memory will be forgotten (Welford 1958). In addition, older adults may assimilate information in smaller units (Obusek & Warren 1973) and accumulate more redundant information (Rabbitt 1977).

Finally, this discussion would not be complete without reference to compensatory strategies (Perlmutter 1988). Older adults are actively involved in adapting to declining abilities. Birren (1969) found that older individuals were keenly aware of the need for conserving time and resources and recognized the usefulness of taking advice. It is these adaptive qualities that are typically lost in laboratory research on problem solving; however, they represent some of the more interesting aspects of development during the later years, since humankind is, above all, a strategic animal (Birren & Perlmutter, in press). Already we are faced with convincing evidence that the behavioural aspects of aging cannot be simplified into a metaphor of a simple downhill slide to the end of life.

HIGHER COGNITIVE PROCESSES: METAMEMORY, PROBLEM SOLVING, AND WISDOM

Three areas currently receiving attention are metamemory, problem solving, and wisdom. Lachman and Lachman (1980) described ''knowledge actualization'' as a functional or real-world memory that reflects a lifetime of education and experience. In contrast to research on secondary memory, there were no age differences found in adults' temporal knowledge actualization (Perlmutter et al. 1980) or spatial knowledge (Perlmutter et al. 1981). Other studies reported an age-related improvement in adults' factual knowledge actualization (Botwinick & Storandt 1974; Lachman & Lachman 1980; Permutter 1978). It appears that an older adult's performance on a memory task will depend, to some degree, on the nature of the task. If the task involves utilizing acquired knowledge, age differences in performance will be minimal or may, in fact, favour older adults. If, however, the task involves primarily the use of basic memory processes, older adults show some performance deficits.

One of the important components relevant to successful knowledge actualization is metamemory knowledge (Lachman & Lachman 1980), knowledge about the functioning of the memory system itself. This knowledge is thought to be particularly important in assisting individuals in selecting strategies that will significantly enhance performance. The investigation of metamemory and its contribution to memory performance is still in the early stages. There remains the question of how to define operationally and assess metamemory, and the nature of the relationship between memory and metamemory (Cavanaugh & Perlmutter 1982).

Some of the monitoring tasks indicative of an individual's ability to use memory knowledge are memory prediction, confidence rating, and feeling-of-knowledge judgments. Preliminary data seem to show stability in performance on monitoring tasks across the life span. Perlmutter (1978) compared a group of older adults, mean age 62 years, and a group of young adults, mean age of 23 years, and reported no age differences in their level of accuracy at predicting recall or recognition responses. Similarly, Perlmutter

(1978) and Lachman and Lachman (1980) reported no age differences in adults' accuracy in making "feeling-of-knowledge" judgments. This implies that young and old adults are comparable in their ability to monitor memory and that age differences in memory are not attributable to differences in monitoring skills.

Various types of tasks have been developed to study the process of skilled problem solving. Among these are concept formation and transformation tasks. The latter involves transporting a given number of elements from one point to another under a certain set of restrictions (Stafford 1983). More commonly used are concept formation tasks, which require subjects to identify a rule that permits them to sort complex objects into a number of specified or prescribed subsets. While it is beyond the scope of this paper to describe these tasks in detail, successful performance depends on learning and memorizing rules and organizing this material so that it can be recalled and used in conjunction with new information to arrive at a successful solution.

Charness (1981) maintained that two sources of age differences exist: changes in the "hardware" of the organism and those in the "software." The hardware of the organism includes short-term memory, long-term memory, working memory, and speed of behaviour. These are relatively invariant processing mechanisms in comparison to the software, those organizational strategies and devices actively utilized by the organism to increase problem-solving ability.

An interesting finding by Stafford (1983) suggested that there are significant age differences in the effects of practice on performance of a transformation task. While young adults were able to improve their performance with practice, as measured by the mean number of moves to solution, practice failed to improve the performance of older adults. There was, however, a great deal of variability in the performance of older adults. With practice, young adults made more errors at points closer to the final goal, while older adults continued throughout the trials to make errors at early subgoals in the solution. This suggests that older adults are less able to determine an efficient progression of subgoals which will ultimately achieve the final goal. In addition, older adults in the study generally took longer to complete the task than young adults. This age difference remained relatively stable across the trials. Although hardware components were not specifically measured in this study, it is likely that age differences can be accounted for, in part, by a hypothesis of age-related behavioural slowing (Birren et al. 1980). This study, however, supports the idea of deficits in the software components of working memory and strategy utilization.

The concept of wisdom has an extensive history and is typically associated with development in old age. It is, however, a relatively unstudied area for reasons which include the absence of good operational definitions and the absence of behavioural criteria to distinguish the wise from the unwise. Clayton and Birren (1980) found that wisdom is perceived as an integration of general cognitive, affective, and reflective qualities. When three cohorts – young, middle-aged, and older adult – were compared there was general agreement that the reflective component, characterized by the qualities of introspection and intuition, and the affective component, characterized by the qualities of understanding, empathy, peacefulness, and gentleness, were integral to the concept of wisdom. In addition, all age groups identified an age-related or developmental component of wisdom.

In the above study, cohort differences emerged in the cognitive structure of wisdom. Older adults identified time-dependent qualities (for example, knowledge and experience), which were not necessarily age-related, and the cognitive qualities of intellect, pragmatism, and observation. A particularly interesting finding was that younger adults were more likely to associate wisdom with age while older adults were less accepting of this positive age-related stereotype. Older adults did not perceive a relationship between their own aging process and wisdom. In addition, they did not judge themselves as having more or less wisdom than other age groups. In contrast to the younger group, older adults perceived understanding and empathy as being more similar to wisdom than were chronological age or experience. Clayton and Birren (1980) suggested that future research should focus on how wisdom is related to species survival, the universal and culture-specific features of wisdom, and the way in which wisdom is achieved across the life span.

PERSONALITY: STABILITY AND CHANGE

It has been suggested that personality is the most significant factor in adaptation to aging (Costa & McCrae 1980; Neugarten 1977). Research in this area addresses two major questions: the extent to which aging affects personality and the way in which personality affects the life situation in old age.

Personality research is characterized by diverse theoretical orientations and methods, which inevitably have led to great differences in empirical findings. Psychoanalytic theory defines personality as a system of dynamic and sometimes conflicting drives and forces and adaptive mechanisms. Perhaps the most prominent theorist from this orientation to address the later stages of development was Erikson (1959, 1963), who suggested that successful aging is characterized by ego integrity, the feeling that one's life has been worthwhile and meaningful. Psychoanalytic constructs, such as ego integrity, are difficult to operationalize, thus limiting rigorous empirical investigation of existing theory. Social psychologists such as Mischel (1968) argued against the stability of personality traits across situations and suggested that behaviour can best be understood by looking at the interaction between person and environment. Role theorists look to prevailing social conditions, including stereotypes of aging and social roles assigned to the elderly, to explain personality change over the life span.

Costa and McCrae (1976) compared personality structure in groups of young, middle-aged, and old males using a cluster analytic approach. Age differences were not found on two dimensions of personality, anxiety-adjustment and introversion-extroversion. In contrast, other studies have suggested an age-related trend towards introversion-extraversion (Schaie & Parham 1976; Thomae 1980). During recent years, however, methodological problems arising from different research designs and sampling from widely disparate populations have made comparison difficult and may account for the contradictory nature of the evidence. A third dimension, openness to experience, revealed between-group differences in which young subjects showed openness to feelings, middle-aged subjects showed openness to ideas, and older subjects showed openness to both feelings and ideas.

There is considerable clinical evidence attesting to the stability of personality (Costa & McCrae 1980). In their sample of middle-aged men, Costa and McCrae (1978) found that most subjects perceived no significant changes in their personality over the past ten years. Coping styles appear to be relatively stable throughout adulthood (Reichard et al. 1962). Longitudinal studies, although few in number, provide further evidence for the continuity of personality across the life span (Britton & Britton 1972, Costa et al. 1980; Leon et al. 1979; Siegler et al. 1979). In general, longitudinal and sequential studies show greater stability in personality than cross-sectional studies. Schaie and Parham (1976), in a sequential study of individuals 21–84 years of age, reported more stability than change in personality measures. The trait of rigidity has been shown to increase with age in cross-sectional designs; however, using a cross-sequential design, Schaie and Strother (1968) suggested that age-related increases in rigidity were due primarily to cultural rather than maturational factors. Similarly, in a follow-up study of college students who were retested twenty-five years after initial testing and compared to a new group of students, cohort differences were found to be greater than age differences (Woodruff & Birren, 1972).

Recent studies from Gothenburg, Sweden, tend to corroborate the longitudinal evidence for stability across the life span. Nilsson (1983) gathered both cross-sectional and longitudinal data from individuals 50–79 years of age. A comparison between 50- and 70-year-olds showed significantly lower extraversion scores for the older group. Among women, 70-year-olds scored higher on neuroticism than 50--year-olds. Berg (1980) also found that women reported less psychological well-being in old age, which is in accord with the finding of Bengtson et al. (1977) that the experience of old age may be significantly different in the two sexes and more difficult for women than men because of the related factors of longer life expectancy, the greater likelihood of being widowed, and the high incidence of women living alone during the later years. Although Nilsson (1983) also found these cross-sectional differences, there were no intraindividual differences in a longitudinal comparison between 75- and 79-year-olds.

Similar results were reported by Nilsson and Persson (1983, 1984). A sample of 70-year-old men and women in Gothenburg was followed up at ages 75 and 79 to determine the extent of personality change. The Marke Nyman Temperament Scale was used to assess the dimensions of validity, solidity, and stability. Only minimal changes were demonstrated, and these included small decreases in personal involvement in men and mental energy in women. Between ages 75 and 79, there was an increase in the tendency for dissociation in men. Also among men, a low level of mental energy at age 70 was related to increased mortality (Nilsson & Persson 1983).

A later study (Nilsson & Persson 1984) investigated different traits using the Cesarec Marke Personality Schedule, which measures various psychogenic needs as defined by Murray. The findings of this study also identified minimal changes among a sample of 70-year-olds, followed up at ages 75 and 79. Although no changes were found for most needs, there was a small increase in the need for order and conformity among both men and women. Among women there was a tendency toward lower need for exhibition, dominance, and aggressive non-conformity and higher succorance. Among men, a higher need for defence of status and lower needs for exhibition and dominance at age 70 were related to increased mortality. Nilsson and Persson (1983, 1984) suggested that cross-sectional analyses would have provided quite a different and misleading picture of personality development among these older adults.

Therefore, the bulk of the literature suggests that personality development during the later years is characterized by stability rather than change. When changes have been reported, they have been minimal and primarily involved decreases in extroversion. In comparison to cross-sectional designs, sequential or longitudinal designs appear to portray a more realistic view of the stability of personality with age.

MODELS AND METAPHORS OF AGING

The previous discussion presented us with a picture of the aging individual as typically being relatively stable in personality while showing a diversity of differences in cognitive abilities. There is, concurrent with an increase in knowledge and skills, a slowness of behaviour. When we add to this equation the problems that some people experience with vision, hearing, and movement, a very complex picture of aging emerges. There is in the picture a stable observer whose values do not shift much over the adult span, one who has evolved strategies to deal with environmental demands and personal needs. One of the realizations that accompanies this picture is that our concepts of contemporary science are very limited.

Aging, from the point of view of science, is at present a collection of many particulars, many islands of knowledge without many bridges. Micro theories derived from specialties within disciplines have guided most of the research. There is therefore a scarcity of conceptualizations that can help the modern person understand his or her aging. Slow to emerge alongside the rapid development of empirical research on aging have been concepts and theory. One might plausibly hold the view that prescientific concepts of aging are alive and flourishing.

Gruman (1966) reviewed ideas about aging and prolongation of life that were prevalent prior to 1800, the beginning of the scientific era. While humankind's wish for immortality has since been recast in many forms, beliefs in healing waters, secret formulas, and mystical forces are still commonplace today. The informed person depends on scientific information about the benefits of avoiding excessive drinking, exercising, controlling stress and not smoking, yet these pockets of data are woven into a picture blended with myth and supposition to compensate for the fact that science is at any stage incomplete and that the science of aging in particular is at an early stage. Were the issue a question about the organization of the universe, we could defer the matter to the future to answer. But human aging is at the same time so pervasive and so personal a topic that we all must have some views and opinions about it.

This century's longer life expectancy and the accelerating growth of the older population have brought with them many challenges to the ideas underlying our institutions and expressed in our social ethics about the proper and fair way to deal with persons in need as well as those whose lives can only be maintained with high technology while there appears to be no awareness of existence. Gruman stated this appropriately: "the modern era has been characterized by a marked decline of faith in supernatural salvation from death, i.e., immortality and resurrection by divine fiat. While these beliefs still are adhered to by many in times of bereavement, their role in everyday life has been weakened greatly, and attention has become centered on the things of this world, especially on the increasing production and distribution of goods and services. Yet, despite the material satisfactions of modern life, the individual feels hollow and powerless when faced by death" (Gruman 1966, p 5).

Growing old in the postindustrial society can be ambiguous. Life expectancy has been dramatically extended while the work life has been shortened by earlier retirement for many. The aging society has brought with it new uncertainties about how individuals find meaning in their lives and how the different age groups establish a fair distribution of resources in society, that is, generational equity. In this century we have become dependent on information provided by the scientific community to guide our decisions in many aspects of life. Our dependence upon science in our search for understanding the unknown has been extended, reasonably, to our attempt to understand aging. Yet science offers only probabilities at present, some with large errors of estimate, and less certainty than we might find comfortable when we raise questions about the meaning of a long life and how phenomena of aging are organized.

Few topics have greater implications than aging. Aging is not only an area of scientific interest but also a heavily value-laden area of personal and social concern (Pifer & Bronte 1986). There are many scientific concepts and metaphors used at present that are carry-overs from previous eras. As we have noted, the scientific era in thought about aging essentially began in the last century and we still face the legacy of those deeply entrenched beliefs about aging (Gruman 1966).

While biological scientists have been preoccupied with the increasing vulnerability of organisms with age, social scientists have devoted attention to the social roles we play and how these change with age. The latter have also concerned themselves with the age grading of status and age norms of behaviour, as well as the relationship of age to morale and life satisfaction (Butt & Beiser 1987). These studies involve those aspects of human life that are socially determined, that is, age characteristics that are the result of the social structure of the society in which individuals grow up and grow old. Since status is arbitrarily bestowed on individuals by a society, it is neither inherently incremental nor decremental with time but reflects the values of the society.

In contrast to biological and social theories of aging, psychological theories explain individual differences. There appear to be wide differences in many behavioural characteristics with age (Birren & Schaie 1985). The influences that give rise to individual differences presumably involve different explanations than the universal behaviours that all humans show over wide ranges of environmental difference. The evolution of a large brain appears to carry with it the capacity to intervene in the way in which we age. We discuss more fully later the relevance of the evolution of the human capacity to plan and develop strategies. Without an active organism, however, such strategies are equivalent to the software of a computer programmed to control events. The active organism uses these strategies to put an imprint on change as it strives to maintain a dynamic equilibrium with its environment.

Some of our capacities appear to decline with age and others seem to improve or at least remain indifferent to age. Our desire to venerate older individuals for their past contributions to society may not run parallel to their current behavioural capacities. It is even less clear how capacities can run contrary paths with age. How can one show increments and decrements in behaviour at the same time that biological viability is declining and social status may be either increasing or decreasing? How can we describe the aging of such a complex system when variability is so great?

AGE AND THE ORGANIZATION OF NATURAL PHENOMENA: TIME DIRECTION AND AGING

"Time is the messenger of the gods that passes without restraint through space, matter, and minds" (Birren & Cunningham 1985). This metaphorical statement is intended to emphasize the importance and the pervasiveness of time in all phenomena. To the above statement we might add that time also passes without restraint through our societies. The placing of events in a time sequence is basic to our concepts of causality. Any organization that is said to *age* must have direction in time. Time is closely linked to the direction of events which lead either to increased disorder (entropy) or to the opposite, increased order (negentropy).

What then is aging? Is there a phase in life in which the organism begins to lose its capacity for self-organization, a phase in which it moves from order to disorder, towards increased entropy and away from negentropy? Although during the later adult years of life the probability of dying increases as a consequence of the organism's decreasing biological capacity for self-regulation, one can observe an orderly maturation of the individual in which early biological capacity for self-regulation is followed by achieving social and, later still, psychological self-regulation.

One international scientist concerned with direction of time is Stephen Hawking. As a consequence of a degenerative disease of the nervous system, he has been confined to a wheelchair. In 1986 he gave a speech. No longer able to speak, he typed his address into a computer mounted on his wheelchair; the speech was then delivered by a synthesizer with an artificial voice. Here we clearly see support systems providing increased energy and information to maintain him in the face of biological decrement, while at another level he was attempting to supply negentropy through his thoughts about the direction of time in the universe. This example illustrates the fact that there is a loose coupling between biological time and psychological time. Perhaps, up to a point, the arrows of time – the thermodynamic arrow and the psychological arrow – may move in different directions. Of note in the example of Hawking's behaviour is that he was generating information at one level while he was losing information at another.

For some aged persons, biological, psychological, and social dynamics may be such that only the most fragile equilibrium can be sustained and information, energy, and affection must be made available lest these individuals become distressed and uncomfortable and die before their time. For some in the later years, we may debate whether the level of life is so fragile and unknowing that the termination of life-support systems should be considered. Others in whom the blend of elements is more favourable may be encouraged to reach for higher goals, and be urged to set their hurdle levels one notch higher in intellectual, physical, or emotional functioning.

NOVEL STRATEGIES: ADAPTATION AND TRANSCENDENCE

The evolution of modern science brings with it an enlarged capacity for strategies whereby we can transcend our earlier limits to biological self-regulation and become that which we were not, for example, a species which has the capacity to overcome the toxic effects of viruses it never met during the course of its evolution. We as a species have also exposed ourselves to environments which we have never met before, such as the weightless state in space: this points to our ability to strategically and creatively override our biological and social limitations.

One area in which we can exercise creativity and strategic override is in our attitudes toward ourselves. How do we regard ourselves in relation to age? What are our self-concept, self-esteem, and related aspirations? These influence how we deploy ourselves. Some strategies involve the maintenance and expansion of the concept of self, which is correlated with good mental health and survival, let alone matters of social productivity and life satisfaction (Tyler 1978). For example, one strategy would be to uncouple the concept of aging from that of disease, accentuating aging as a natural, intrinsic, and *normal* part of life that requires some preparation to be fully enjoyed. A further strategy would be to extend the view that aging, in addition to being a normal part of life, has some meaning of its own.

Humankind is entering an era of the aging society, a society in which we are living longer, working shorter, and having fewer children (Pifer & Bronte 1986). Our values are in many instances appropriate to earlier eras but continue by inertia into the present, confusing the fact that new phenomena of aging are emerging. Our law courts are increasingly attending to matters of age discrimination, forced retirement, guardianship, conservatorship, and other issues related to aging. These court hearings help to sharpen the issues of fact as well as our feelings about the facts and what is viewed as just and fair in a changing society. The issues of aging are so complex that each generation may offer its own primary metaphors about it, with individuals sharing in the pool of common metaphor while searching for their personal ones. We have an obligation to use our capacities and to trade in and trade up our old metaphors in response to new data gathered by scientists.

Studying autobiographies impresses one with the great capacity humankind has for adapting to environmental circumstances and events (Birren & Hedlund 1987). If we were merely showing plastic adaptability, such as the reptile displays by reducing activity in cold weather, it would be less dramatic than the fact that we have strategic adaptability. Unlike the adaptations that have been built into less complex species by selective pressures and that are encoded in their DNA, our nervous systems permit strategic and novel adaptations as well. Thus, while an older individual may show a restricted range of adaptability to the environment because of a diminished capacity for biological self-regulation, and while he or she may lose vital social support networks from earlier years, this same individual may continue to obviate these limitations by effective strategies. It is here that the concept of wisdom needs to be introduced: the capacity of an individual to take into account physical limitations and social circumstances, giving rise to a superordinating control that extends the capacity for self-regulation beyond the previous bounds. Such persons contribute to the frustration of the empirical scientist who attempts to extrapolate from experimental studies and predict the competence of an individual in "real life." Some individuals expand their effectiveness and capacity for self-regulation in the presence of major decreases in internal and external resources until a short interval in late life, the phase of terminal decline.

Our self-regard and self-esteem are influenced by what we do about caring for dependent older persons and about the circumstances surrounding them at the end of their lives. Human groups are noted for their tendency to develop rituals surrounding the dying and the dead. Some believe that if they fail to take care of the dying and to respect the dead appropriately, the spirits of the departed may blight their lives. By personal projection, the dying and the dead are part of ourselves and we are treating a part of us in our care and rituals. Robert Anderson (1970), at the end of his play *I Never Sang for My Father,* made the point that death may end a life but not the relationship. The relationships we have had with others live on in terms of their influences. It is not surprising, therefore, that a mystique develops about the care of the dependent aged and the circumstances of their deaths. It is not easy to neglect the care of the elderly without at the same time neglecting our self-concept, and it is not easy to wish for the death of a family member without at the same time wishing for a partial death of oneself.

Death is a major aspect of life, onto which we project our uncertainties, fantasies, fears, and unresolved ambitions. It is not unreasonable that most religions have some tenets about the aged, as they do about death itself. Religious institutions commonly have a role in managing and expressing our thoughts about aging, the care of the aged, and dying. Scientific advances and humanistic enlightenment have not lessened our need for creativity in developing systems of faith. Wagar (1971) said: "Man. . . suddenly found himself living in a post-ideological, anti-utopian, demythologized world in which the will to believe had withered and failed." One issue needing attention is whether an empirical ideology can suffice to maintain the self-respect and productivity of individuals and societies as they grow old. Aging is too important to leave to the scientists, but it is also too important to leave to the theologians and humanists. From all of these and from our own experiences will come the creative metastrategies that will enable us to transcend the limitations that grow more probable as we grow older.

These are matters about which science has little to say directly. Science can best be relied upon to give accurate descriptions of "what is" and, with somewhat less fidelity, can give us descriptions of "what can be." But ethics and the humanities are more commonly concerned with "what should be." The creation of systems of thought that deal with goals and related prescriptions is not an area in which science plays its strongest role. Since the subject of aging reminds all of us of our mortality, perhaps we can use it to promote a useful dialogue between the sciences and humanities. In this way we may encourage societies of intelligent and wise individuals to build cultures that are not only technologically advanced but also humane.

The thesis of this paper is that our aging is a product of many complex forces. Our wisdom and our metastrategies can be brought to bear directly on the issue of how we want to grow old. Only through examination of our scientific metaphors and through interdisciplinary exchange between humanists and scientists can theory in aging progress. Only through these can our ethical behaviour in caring for the dependent elderly and caring about the circumstances of their death develop.

REFERENCES

Anderson, R. (1970). *I never sang for my father*. New York: Signet

Bengtson, V.L., Kasschau, P.L., Ragan, P.K. (1977). The impact of social structure on aging individuals. In J.E. Birren and K.W. Schaie (Eds.), *Handbook of the psychology of aging*. New York: Van Nostrand Reinhold

Berg, S. (1980). Psychological functioning in 70 and 75 year old people: A study in an industrialized city. *Acta Psychiatrica Scandinavica Supplementum, 228,* 63

Birren, J.E. (1969). Age and decision strategies. In A.T. Welford and J.E. Birren (Eds.), *Interdisciplinary topics in gerontology* (Vol. 4). Basel: S. Karger

Birren, J.E., & Cunningham, W.R. (1985). Research on the psychology of aging. In J.E. Birren and K.W. Schaie (Eds.), *Handbook of the psychology of aging*. New York: Van Nostrand Reinhold

Birren, J.E., & Hedlund, B. (1987). Contributions of autobiography to developmental psychology. In N. Eisenberg (Ed.), *Contemporary topics in developmental gerontology*. New York: John Wiley & Sons

Birren, J.E., & Perlmutter, M. (in press). Measuring our psychological performance. In R.N. Butler (Ed.), *The promise of productive aging*. New York: Springer

Birren, J.E. & Schaie, W.K. (1985). *Handbook of the psychology of aging*. New York: Van Nostrand Reinhold

Birren, J.E., & Schroots, J.J.F. (1980). Aging, from cell to society: A search for new metaphors. Paper presented at the World Health Organizational Meeting, Mexico City

Birren, J.E., Woods, A.M., & Williams, M.V. (1980). Behavioral slowing with age: Causes, organization, and consequences. In L.W. Poon (Ed.), *Aging in the 1980s: Psychological issues*. Washington, DC: American Psychological Association

Botwinick, J. (1966). Cautiousness in advanced age. *J. Geront., 21,* 347–53

Botwinick, J., & Storandt, M. (1974). *Memory, related functions, and age*. Springfield, IL: Charles C. Thomas

Britton, J.H., & Britton, J.O. (1972). *Personality changes in aging: A longitudinal study of community residence*. New York: Springer

Butt, S.D., & Beiser, M. (1987). Successful aging: A theme for international psychology. *Psychology and Aging, 2,* 87–94

Cavanaugh, J.C., & Perlmutter, M. (1982). Metamemory: A critical examination. *Child Development, 53,* 11–28

Charness, N. (1981). Aging and skilled problem-solving. *Journal of Experimental Psychology: General, 110,* 21–38

Clayton, V.P., & Birren, J.E. (1980). The development of wisdom across the life-span: A reexamination of an ancient topic. In P.B. Baltes and O.G. Brim, Jr. (Eds.), *Life span development and behavior* (Vol. 3). New York: Academic Press

Comfort, A. (1956). *The biology of senescence*. London: Routledge & Kegan Paul

Costa, P.T., & McCrae, R.R. (1976). Age differences in personality structure: A cluster analytic approach. *Journal of Gerontology, 31,* 564–70

Costa, P.T., & McCrae, R.R. (1978). Objective personality assessment. In M. Storandt, I.C. Siegler, and M.F. Elias (Eds.), *The clinical psychology of aging*. New York: Plenum

Costa, P.T., McCrae, R.R., & Arenberg, D. (1980). Dispositions in adult males. *Journal of Personality and Social Psychology, 38,* 793–800

Erikson, E.H. (1959). *Identity and the life cycle: Psychological issues, 1*. New York: International Universities Press

Erikson, E.H. (1963). *Childhood and society* (2nd ed.) New York: W.W. Norton

Gardner, E.F., & Monge, R.H. (1977). Adult age differences in cognitive abilities and educational background. *Experimental Aging Research,* 337–83

Gruman, G.J. (1966). *A history of ideas about the prolongation of life: The evolution of prolongevity hypotheses to 1800*. Philadelphia: American Philosophical Society

Handler, P. (1960). Radiation and aging. In N.W. Shock (Ed.), *Aging,* 199–223. Washington, DC: Government Printing Office

Lachman, J.L., & Lachman, R. (1980). Age and the actualization of world knowledge. In L.W. Poon, J.L. Fozard, L.S. Cermak, D. Arenberg, and L.W. Thompson (Eds.), *New directions in memory and aging: Proceedings of the George A. Thailand Memorial Conference*. Hillsdale, NJ: Lawrence Erlbaum Associates

Lansing, A.I. (1959). General biology of senescence. In J.E. Birren (Ed.), *Handbook of aging and the individual,* 119–35. Chicago: University of Chicago Press

Leon, G.R., Gillum, B., Gillum, R., & Gouze, M. (1979). Personality stability and change over a 30-year period: Middle age to older age. *Journal of Consulting and Clinical Psychology, 47,* 517–24

Mischel, W. (1968). *Personality and assessment*. New York: Wiley & Sons

Neugarten, B.L. (1977). Personality and aging. In J.E. Birren and K.W. Schaie (Eds.), *Handbook of the psychology of aging*. New York: Van Nostrand Reinhold

Nilsson, L.V. (1983). Personality changes in the aged: A transactional and longitudinal study with the Eysenck Personality Inventory. *Acta Psychiatrica Scandinivica 68,* 141–418

Nilsson, L.V., & Persson, G. (1984). Personality changes in the aged: A longitudinal study of psychogenic needs with the CMPS. *Acta Psychiatrica Scandinivica 69,* 182–89

Obusek, C.J., & Warren, R.M. (1973). Comparison of speech perception in senile and well-preserved aged by means of the verbal transformation effect. *Journal of Gerontology, 28,* 188–98

Perlmutter, M. (1978). What is memory aging the aging of? *Developmental Psychology, 14,* 330–45

Perlmutter, M. (1988). Cognitive potential throughout life. In J.E. Birren and V.L. Bengtson (Eds.), *Emergent theories in aging*. New York: Springer

Perlmutter, M., Metzger, R., Miller, K., & Nezworski, T. (1980). Memory of historical events. *Experimental Aging Research, 6,* 47–60

Perlmutter, M., Metzger, R., Nezworski, T., & Miller, K. (1981). Spatial and temporal memory in 20 and 60 year olds. *Journal of Gerontology, 36,* 59–65

Pifer, A., & Bronte, L. (1986). *Our aging society*. New York: W.W. Norton

Rabbitt, P. (1977). Changes in problem-solving ability in old age. In J.E. Birren and K.W. Schaie (Eds.), *Handbook of the psychology of aging*. New York: Van Nostrand Reinhold

Reichard, S., Livson, F., & Peterson, P.G. (1962). *Aging and personality*. New York: Wiley & Sons

Salthouse, T.A. (1980). Age and memory: Strategies for localizing the loss. In L.W. Poon, J.L. Fozard, L.S. Cermak, D. Zrenberg, and L.W. Thompson (Eds.), *New directions in memory and aging: Proceedings of the George A. Thailand Memorial Conference*. Hillsdale, NJ: Lawrence Erlbaum Associates

Schaie, K.W. (1980). Intelligence and problem solving. In J.E. Birren and R.B. Sloane (Eds.), *Handbook of mental health and aging*. Englewood Cliffs, NJ: Prentice-Hall

Schaie, K.W., & Parham, I.A. (1976). Stability of adult personality traits: Facts or fable? *Journal of Personality and Social Psychology, 34,* 146–58

Schaie, K.W., & Strother, C.R. (1968). Cognitive and personality variables in college graduates of advanced ages. In G.A. Talland (Ed.), *Human aging and behavior*. New York: Academic Press

Siegler, I.C., George, L.K., & Okum, M.A. (1979). A cross-sectional analysis of adult personality. *Developmental Psychology, 15,* 350–51.

Stafford, J.L. (1983). *Skilled problem-solving ability and the effects of practice in young and elderly adults*. Unpublished doctoral dissertation, University of Southern California

Thomae, H. (1980). Personality and adjustment to aging. In J.E. Birren and R.B. Sloane (Eds.), *Handbook of mental health and aging*. Englewood Cliffs, NJ: Prentice-Hall

Tyler, L.E. (1978). *Individuality: Human possibility and personal choice in the psychological development of men and women*. San Francisco: Jossey Bass

Wagar, W.W. (1971). Religion, ideology, and the idea of mankind in contemporary history. In W.W. Wagar (Ed.), *History and the idea of mankind*. Albuquerque, NM: University of New Mexico Press

Welford, A.T. (1958). *Aging and human skill*. Oxford: Oxford University Press

Woodruff, D.S. & Birren, J.E. (1972). Age changes and cohort differences in personality. *Developmental Psychology, 6,* 252–59

6

Cognitive Intervention in Later Life: Philosophical Issues

DAVID F. HULTSCH AND JANE H. MCEWAN

Over the years, we have become increasingly optimistic about the cognitive ability of adults. At a general level, more and more theory and research have been guided by a model which assumes that many of the changes occurring during adulthood are a function of non-universal, extrinsic, and experientially-based processes (Baltes et al. 1984; Denney 1984). This model suggests that such changes are, in principle, preventable or modifiable, given discovery and manipulation of the extrinsic antecedents that control them.

The usefulness of this approach is reflected in a variety of data sets. For example, over the last two decades descriptive research has seriously challenged the validity of findings suggesting a pattern of inevitable general decline of intellectual functioning with increasing age. Rather, these data suggest the importance of generational differences in cognitive functioning, and the role of various health and experiential factors in producing differential patterns of change (Schaie 1979, 1984). At another level, manipulative studies have shown the efficacy of modifying "typical" age functions (Poon 1985; Schaie & Willis 1986). For example, it has been found that instructing subjects to use various encoding and retrieval strategies leads to the attenuation and sometimes elimination of adult age differences in memory performance (Craik 1977). In addition to direct instruction, non-cognitive techniques such as practice, modelling, feedback, and others have been demonstrated to result in improvements in the performance of older adults on a variety of cognitive tasks (Denney 1979). Such findings do not point to the absence of age-related declines in cognitive functioning. However, they do suggest the existence of considerable interindividual variation and potential for growth (plasticity).

Coinciding with this increasing optimism concerning the cognitive adaptability of adults have been many other more generic developments, including concern for minority groups, the projected aging of our population, and the increasing rate of social change. The confluence of these factors has led to greater emphasis on programmatic intervention in general and interest in "redesigning the aging process" (Kastenbaum 1968) in particular, from the modification of age-grading in society (Schaie 1973), to lifelong education in all of its manifestations (Birren & Woodruff 1973; Willis 1985).

Although we have the technology to alter many behavioural manifestations of aging, we still need to consider carefully the assumptions underlying such intervention efforts. For example, we have frequently assumed that older adults are deprived and have used this as a rationale for intervention. However, it is not a simple concept. One may distinguish between objective and sensed deprivation. Sensed deprivation, in turn, may be differentiated into relative and subjective deprivation. Relative deprivation involves an invidious comparison between a person and an explicit reference group, whereas subjective deprivation involves an invidious comparison between one's present status and an habitual, expected, or desired state.

It is quite likely that many elderly suffer from all three types of deprivation (Bortner & Hultsch 1974; NICHD 1968). Yet this fact does not point directly to intervention. For example, if one argues that the poorer cognitive performance of older adults relative to younger adults is evidence for relative deprivation, does this justify efforts to modify the behaviour of older people to conform to that of the younger, reference group? This approach assumes that the behaviours exhibited by older adults are dysfunctional while those exhibited by younger ones are functional. The problem is similar to that raised in connection with various minority groups (Tulkin 1972). Such efforts run the risk of ignoring cultural relativism and neglecting political and social realities which may be partly responsible for the differences in the first place. The point is that there are many considerations involved in programmatic intervention efforts beyond the technology necessary to accomplish them. The purpose of this paper is to explore some of the philosophical and moral issues which must be considered before we design and implement interventions in the field of aging.

THE PHILOSOPHY OF INTERVENTION

It may be useful at the outset to consider the multiple components of the intervention process itself (Jacobs 1972). One can identify at least three aspects: decision content, decision referents and decision makers. First, there are multiple decisions related to the content of the intervention process. These include goals (alleviation, enrichment, prevention), target behaviours (intellectual abilities, personality traits, specific knowledge, attitudes), mechanisms (practice, psychotherapy, environmental change), agents (professionals, paraprofessionals), order (priorities, timing), and setting (laboratory, classroom, hospital, community). Second, there are different aspects of program implementation; for example, research and development, service delivery, training, and program evaluation. Finally, it is important to note that decisions about these aspects of the intervention process are made by many individuals at several different levels (Rappaport 1977). These range from the larger society itself, through elected officials, regulatory agencies, program specialists and program staff, to the clientele of the intervention. Intervention decisions, then, do not flow directly from what we know about a particular phenomenon. In part, our awareness of the problem, ability to generate alternative solutions, and ability to predict outcomes are limited by the quality and accuracy of information available. At the same time, the selection of information and the choices made about how to proceed are very much influenced by multiple value systems. The very notion of intervention presupposes both a dimension of "quality of functioning" and value judgments about the target of intervention as compared to that criterion. Thus, there is no such thing as an evaluatively or ethically neutral intervention. As Chandler (1980) has pointed out, if we lack a defensible value orientation, we cannot say that one way of being is better or worse than another. Moreover, "quality of functioning" can be examined on a continuum ranging from the individual level to the societal level, and the well-being of any unit on that scale can arbitrarily be given priority.

Whose Goals are Being Realized?

As noted above, intervention decisions are made at multiple levels, such as those of federal and municipal governments and social service agencies. These decisions reflect the goals of various individuals (especially those with power and influence), groups, and segments of the social structure. Whenever more than one decision-maker is involved in the development, implementation, and evaluation of an intervention program, conflict may arise. For example, the province of British Columbia funds inpatient and outpatient treatment programs for alcohol abuse (intervention at the individual level, to ameliorate dysfunction), *and* employs merchandising strategies intended to increase impulse buying in government-operated liquor stores (intervention at the governmental level, to increase revenues). Similarly, conflict may be created if more than one group is affected, either directly or indirectly, by the intervention. For example, it may be seen as both humane and socially responsible for the government to provide medical services such as prescription drugs, wheelchairs, and eyeglasses free of charge to indigent seniors. Yet some of the physically healthy, non-indigent taxpayers may complain if their taxes are increased (or if subsidies to recreation centres are reduced) in order to cover the cost of such services.

The impact of the decision-maker tends to decrease as one moves down the list – that is, from society to clientele. An important issue here is that since the clients (or targets) of intervention are seldom consulted about *their* goals, the designers and implementors of intervention programs may end up imposing their own values on the targets. Even if the goal of intervention is to improve "quality of life" (certainly an admirable goal), it is often the intervenor's definition of such quality which is employed as the standard foisted on the targets. This puts the targets in a one-down position, that of being an involuntary client, since they have been told "we know what's best for you (and you don't), and we're giving it to you (even if you don't want it)." Such well-intentioned imperialism can occur with specific health issues, such as fluoridation of the water supply, and with broader issues, such as redesigning the aging process.

Who Should Make Decisions About Goals To Be Supported?

Aging is a natural process which occurs in everyone who does not die "prematurely." By redesigning this process, we could be tinkering with the timing of aging events and of death itself. Might we be inadvertently forcing unwanted changes ("optimization" or "amelioration") on subjects? What if they do not want to have this natural process redesigned? Just as large numbers of women have, during the past twenty years, opted for "natural" childbirth with a minimum of technological intervention, perhaps elders would like to choose the amount of intervention they are willing to accept in their aging process. Who, then, should be charged with making decisions about which goals will be supported? Should it be government officials, professionals who have specialized knowledge of the aging process, or older persons themselves? Clearly, these multiple constituencies must all be involved.

Brandstädter (1980) suggests that psychologists can provide valuable input into the decision-making process in two ways. First, they can assess the feasibility and compatibility of proposed goals. Because of their understanding of individual differences, they can judge what is feasible for each individual; otherwise, we would be wasting resources and annoying the targets of intervention. The compatibility of multiple goals is determined by the feasibility of aggregate goals. Are they simultaneously realizable? Second, psychologists can make "convergent predictions" about the projected efficiency of an intervention, and "divergent predictions" about its possible adverse consequences or side-effects.

What Is the Goal of Intervention?

Age-related changes are perceived and interpreted within the frame of reference provided by our value system. It is probably reasonable to suggest that our culture views aging as a process of decrement and deprivation. Aging is seen as synonymous with physical and intellectual decline, personal and social inadequacy, and economic and cultural deprivation. Even given an optimistic position concerning the modifiability of these decrements, such a view of aging has led to an emphasis on alleviation as a goal. This very notion of intervention suggests that there is something about the target individuals, either now or in the future, which is somehow unacceptable and therefore needs to be changed. We see this with primary intervention, where we try to prevent the development of a disorder or forestall a natural concomitant of increased age; with secondary intervention, where we provide treatment for a disorder, such as programs to improve memory; and with tertiary intervention, where the targets are rehabilitated in order to adjust to their condition.

In evaluating the aging process and its concomitants, we often use the behaviour of young adults as the criterion for optimum functioning. What does this say about our attitudes toward elders and toward the aging process itself? How would we evaluate aging (and, accordingly, design interventions) if the behaviour of older adults were the criterion to be met by younger people? If we move away from the notion of evaluation and view age differences in functioning as merely stylistic (for example, age differences in strategies for remembering word lists), we may have reason to question our intervention goals. If a group's performance is compared to an evaluative standard and found only to be "different," and not "worse," then how do we justify our attempts to change that group's style of performance?

The concept of "differential aging" is frequently ignored when interventions are designed for individuals and groups. This concept suggests that developmental functions show increasing interindividual variability with age, that development is modifiable, and therefore that some age-related changes are reversible. Rather than being unidirectional, psychological aging is both multidirectional and plastic. The important implication here is that intervention should be differential rather than normative, because the pathways of development and aging will differ across behavioural variables and across individuals.

Because we lack a psychological definition of optimal aging, we also lack a coherent set of goals for the intervention process. Is the ideal aged state reflected in life satisfaction, cognitive performance, social utility, or a subjective measure of "quality of life"? While some of these indicators may be readily quantified, especially if we use younger adults as a standard of comparison, the more subjective or value-laden outcomes are harder to assess. Even where measurement instruments exist, for example, life satisfaction inventories, the correlations among them may be weak. This raises the question of how we will know when the goal of (optimization) intervention has been achieved, if we lack a reliable measure of the intended outcome.

Who Is the Target of Intervention?

As Pickett (1980) has pointed out, developmental intervention is often aimed at those who have little power, namely children and the elderly. We are hard-pressed to find a research example of aging intervention in which the target is young adults. It may be argued that our negative view of aging has been a major cause of this problem. Work on early childhood education showed the same value orientation (that is, that children are the ones needing to be ameliorated), and yet significant efforts have been made in this field in recent years to involve the clientele, particularly the parents, in the intervention process. To date, gerontologists have made little effort in this direction; we have not looked at changing the attitudes and behaviour of other age groups or of society as a means of altering the aging process. Neither have we looked at the possibility of changing various parts of the social structure, such as racial, occupational and socio-economic stratification, as alternatives to changing groups.

Kuypers and Bengtson (1973) present a model of normal aging based on the social breakdown syndrome. This model suggests that an individual's sense of self and society are a function of the kinds of social labelling and valuing he or she experiences. The authors suggest that the elderly are susceptible to the social breakdown syndrome because of the role loss, deficient normative information, and lack of reference groups that tend to accompany aging in our culture. This susceptibility leads to an excessive dependence on external cues, which, in the case of the elderly, are essentially negative. Thus, the individual is introduced into a "sick role," and behaviours appropriate to the role are learned while those inappropriate to it are extinguished. The final step is psychological identification and self-labelling as unintelligent, useless, sick, and so on. Studies by Langer and her colleagues (Avorn & Langer 1982; Rodin & Langer 1980; Langer 1981) suggest that the social environment may encourage a negative self-concept and behavioural deficits in those individuals who are labelled or treated as though they were incompetent.

Kuypers and Bengtson suggest several points of possible intervention into this cycle. First, such intervention might increase competence by redefining successful social role performance. In our culture, social role performance is largely defined by productivity. The efficacy of modifying society's ability and willingness to continue the elderly in roles which are currently withdrawn from them is, of course, a separate issue. However, from the individual's point of view, an intervention such as lifelong education might well modify the view that competence is defined by productivity. This may mean focusing our interventions on personal-affective target behaviours as well as cognitive ones. That is, such an attitude change will need to rely on many skills typically not considered cognitive, such as introspection, emotional expressiveness, and interpersonal relations. Obviously, this will not be an easy task, since the elderly will reflect our cultural bias toward cognitive activities in education.

Second, such an intervention might increase competence by developing greater feelings of efficacy and internal locus of control. A significant component of adaptability is the feeling that the source of and responsibility for action lies largely within rather than outside the individual – in other words, the feeling that what one does makes a difference in the outcome of events. On the one hand, increased skill would provide a foundation for such feelings. As the individual becomes more skilled, the probability of achieving desired outcomes increases, and feelings of efficacy increase as well. In addition, however, a greater role in the decisionmaking process itself is important. Let us return here to our earlier point concerning the role of the clientele in intervention. The development of intervention programs in which the elderly play a significant role as decisionmakers would enhance the development of feelings of efficacy and internal locus of control.

SYSTEMS ISSUES IN INTERVENTION

Not only is the intervention process a complex system of decisions, but intervention itself represents an intrusive input into an organized network of active and ongoing processes – that is, a system. From this point of view, it is essential to be aware that when one succeeds in modifying the operation of one set of components of a system, one may be simultaneously modifying the operation of other sets of components with which they are interrelated. The ultimate result is not simply the modification of separate components, but modification of the system as a whole. If we fail to take this into account, many pitfalls are possible as we seek to intervene in the development of adults.

Does New Learning Produce Stress?

Theorists such as Selye (1976) tell us that one concomitant of change is always stress. Others have argued that older adults are more susceptible to stress than younger adults for a variety of reasons. Thus, if we naively assume that new learning is good for older adults and implement massive educational intervention programs accompanied by hard-sell techniques to encourage people to become involved in them, we may actually produce negative outcomes for some individuals.

We might generally assume that new learning will produce greater competence, adjustment, and adaptibility. However, is this necessarily the case? For example, Neugarten et al. (1968) report that in the case of some of the individuals they classify as integrated personality types, low social role activity (implying relatively little new learning) is associated with high life satisfaction. In a similar vein, Clark and Anderson (1967) report that old people who did not exhibit or relinquish high levels of achievement motivation were better adjusted and had fewer mental health problems than those showing the opposite pattern. Now clearly there is no simple conclusion to be drawn from these data. For example, it is quite plausible that a lack of new learning leads to adjustment in these instances because our culture does not encourage, and indeed may punish, new learning in older adults.

Matching Interventions and Environments

If we intervene to ameliorate specific aspects of individual functioning, we can inadvertently cause disharmony between the clients and their environment. For example, studies of personal control (Mullins 1982; Strickland 1979) suggest that it is the compatibility between the environment and the client's locus of control that is important in maintaining well-being. Some environments support an internal control orientation, while others support an external orientation. However, if we were to look only at the large number of studies which report a correlation between internality and well-being (for example, Hunter et al. 1980; Ryden 1984), we could design interventions which increase internality but bring individuals into conflict with the demands of their social environment.

Baltes's work on the operant economy in nursing homes (Baltes 1982; Baltes & Reisenzein 1986) shows that the staff of residential settings encourage and reward dependency behaviour among patients, thus suggesting that the social environment can reward and punish specific behaviours of older individuals. Before designing an intervention, we must understand the dynamics of the interpersonal setting in which it will be implemented.

"Side-Effects" of Intervention

Behaviour is determined by multiple variables, but intervention is likely to be univariate. One difficulty may occur in determining whether a change in the target behaviour has been effected. For example, Willems (1973) reports such a potential problem illustrated by a milieu intervention program designed to modify the environment in order to eliminate isolated standing behaviour in a hospital psychiatric ward. In this case, the psychologists succeeded in eliminating the undesirable behaviour from one setting only to discover that it then occurred in a different setting. Had observations of the target behaviour been restricted to one setting of the environment, an erroneous conclusion would have been reached.

A second effect may occur if the attainment of one behaviour precludes or delays another. For example, Kohlberg (1968) has suggested the possibility that cognitive intervention in early childhood may actually interfere with the sequencing of subsequent cognitive development. At a systems level, this effect could be manifested as a trade-off between independence and efficiency; if residents are given independence training so that they take more responsibility for daily personal care, this may have salutary effects on their psychological well-being, but might also disrupt the work habits of institutional staff, or result in reduced efficiency (for example, in terms of how long it takes a hundred physically incapacitated people to feed themselves as opposed to when they are assisted by staff). This brings us back to the basic values question of "whose goals are being supported?"

A third effect may occur if the attainment of one target behaviour leads to modification of other sets of behaviours as well. For example, let us assume that our society implements a massive lifelong education program with economic and social support. Such an intervention is likely to have many potential transfer effects beyond the behaviours targeted by the program itself. Also, such transfer effects will be both positive and negative.

CONCLUSION

Let us conclude by suggesting that we broaden our perspective concerning intervention in the aging process. First, we must recognize that the intervention process itself is a complex system of decisions. As intervention programmes are being considered, the interaction among various decision-makers must be analysed in order to facilitate congruence among the various decision components. Second, we must recognize that intervention represents an intrusion into a system rather than a modification of independent components. It is not a case of merely coping with "side-effects." Rather, we need to understand the complex interdependencies that characterize the phenomena we wish to modify.

As Willems (1973) has pointed out, these considerations may dictate a certain conservatism with regard to intervention. We need a great deal more empirical data and theory that take account of the interdependencies involved. We are not suggesting foregoing intervention efforts to rehabilitate, remediate, or enhance the cognitive functioning of adults. Rather, we are suggesting that we undertake such efforts aware of the fact that these efforts are rooted in value choices and will have multiple outcomes. The ethical aspects of intervention, in this sense, may well outweigh the technical ones.

REFERENCES

Avorn, J., & Langer, E. (1982). Induced disability in nursing home patients: A controlled trial. *Journal of the American Geriatric Society, 30,* 397–400

Baltes, M.M. (1982). Environmental factors in dependency among nursing home residents: A social ecology analysis. In T.A. Wills (Ed.), *Basic processes in helping relationships*. New York: Academic Press

Baltes, M.M. & Reisenzein, R. (1986). The social world in long-term care institutions: Psychosocial control toward dependency? In M.M. Baltes and P.B. Baltes (Eds.), *Psychology of control and aging*. Hillsdale, NJ: Erlbaum

Baltes, P.B., Dittman-Kohli, F., & Dixon, R.A. (1984). New perspectives on the development of intelligence in adulthood: Toward a dual-process conception and a model of selective optimization with comprehension. In P.B. Baltes & O.G. Brim, Jr. (Eds.), *Life-span development and behavior* (Vol. 6). New York: Academic Press

Birren, J.E., & Woodruff, D.S. (1973). Human development over the life span through education. In P.B. Baltes and K.W. Schaie (Eds.), *Life-span developmental psychology: Personality and socialization*. New York: Academic Press

Bortner, R.W., & Hultsch, D.F. (1974). Patterns of subjective deprivation in adulthood. *Developmental Psychology, 10,* 534–45

Brandtstädter, J. (1980). Relationships between life-span developmental theory, research, and intervention: A revision of some stereotypes. In R.R. Turner and H.W. Reese (Eds.), *Life-span developmental psychology: Intervention*. New York: Academic Press

Chandler, M.J. (1980). Life-span intervention as a symptom of conversion hysteria. In R.R. Turner and H.W. Reese (Eds.), *Life-span developmental psychology: Intervention*. New York: Academic Press

Clark, M., & Anderson, B.G. (1967). *Culture and aging*. Springfield, IL: Charles C. Thomas

Craik, F.I.M. (1977). Age differences in human memory. In J.E. Birren and K.W. Schaie (Eds.), *Handbook of the psychology of aging*. New York: Van Nostrand Reinhold

Denney, N.W. (1979). Problem solving in later adulthood: Intervention research. In P.B. Baltes and O.G. Brim, Jr. (Eds.), *Life-span development and behavior* (Vol. 2) New York: Academic Press

Denney, N.W. (1984). A model of cognitive development across the life span. *Developmental Review, 4,* 171–91

Hunter, K.I., Linn, M.W., Harris, R., & Pratt, T.C. (1980). Discriminators of internal-external locus of control orientation in the elderly. *Research on Aging, 2,* 49–60

Jacobs, A. (1972). Strategies of social intervention: Past and future. In A. Jacobs and W. Spradlin (Eds.), *The group as an agent of change*. Chicago: Aldine

Kastenbaum, R. (1968). Perspectives on the development and modification of behavior in the aged: A developmental-field perspective. *The Gerontologist, 8,* 280–83

Kohlberg, L. (1968). Early education: A cognitive-developmental view. *Child Development, 29,* 1013–62

Kuypers, J.A., & Bengtson, V.L. (1973). Social breakdown and competence: A model of normal aging. *Human Development, 16,* 181–201

Langer, E.J. (1981). Old age: An artifact? In J.M. McGaugh and S. Kiesler (Eds.), *Aging: biology and behavior.* New York: Academic Press

Mullins, L.C. (1982). Locus of desired control and patient role among the institutionalized elderly. *Journal of Social Psychology, 116,* 269–76

National Institute of Child Health and Human Development. (1968). *Perspectives on human deprivation: Biological, psychological, and sociological.* Washington, DC: U.S. Public Health Service

Neugarten, B.L., Havighurst, R.J., & Tobin, S.S. (1968). Personality and patterns of aging. In B.L. Neugarten (Ed.), *Middle age and aging.* Chicago: University of Chicago Press

Pickett, G. (1980). The politics of public intervention. In R.R. Turner and H.W. Reese (Eds.), *Life-span developmental psychology: Intervention.* New York: Academic Press

Poon, L.W. (1985). Differences in human memory with aging: Nature, causes, and clinical implications. In J.E. Birren and K.W. Schaie (Eds.), *Handbook of the psychology of aging* (2nd ed.) New York: Van Nostrand Reinhold

Rappaport, J. (1977). *Community psychology: Values, research and action.* New York: Holt, Rinehart, & Winston

Rodin, J., & Langer, E.J. (1980). Aging and labels: The decline of control and the fall of self-esteem. *Journal of Social Issues, 36,* 12–29

Ryden, M.B. (1984). Morale and perceived control in institutionalized elderly. *Nursing Research, 33,* 130–36

Schaie, K.W. (1973). Reflections on paper by Looft, Peterson, and Sparks: Intervention toward an ageless society. *The Gerontologist, 13,* 31–35

Schaie, K.W. (1979). The primary mental abilities in adulthood: An exploration in the development of psychometric intelligence. In P.B. Baltes and O.G. Brim, Jr. (Eds.), *Life-span development and behavior* (Vol. 2). New York: Academic Press

Schaie, K.W. (1984). Midlife influences upon intellectual functioning in old age. *International Journal of Behavioral Development, 7,* 463–78

Schaie, K.W., & Willis, S.L. (1986). Can decline in adult intellectual functioning be reversed? *Developmental Psychology, 22,* 223–32

Selye, H. (1976). *The stress of life* (2nd ed.) New York: McGraw-Hill

Strickland, B.R. (1979). I-E expectancies and cardiovascular functioning. In L.C. Perlmuter and R.A. Monty (Eds.), *Choice and perceived control.* Hillsdale, NJ: Erlbaum

Tulkin, S.R. (1972). An analysis of the concept of cultural deprivation. *Developmental psychology, 6,* 326–39

Willems, E.P. (1973). Behavioral ecology and experimental analysis: Courtship is not enough. In J.R. Nesselroade and H.W. Resse (Eds.), *Life span developmental psychology: Methodological issues.* New York: Academic Press

Willis, S.L. (1985). Towards an educational psychology of the older adult learner. In J.E. Birren and K.W. Schaie (Eds.), *Handbook of the psychology of aging* (2nd ed.). New York: Van Nostrand Reinhold

7

The Calculus of Discrimination: Discriminatory Resource Allocation for an Aging Population

EIKE-HENNER W. KLUGE

INTRODUCTION

One of the most fundamental tenets of Canadian society is the principle of equality: every person is the equal of every other. It goes hand in hand with another principle which we consider equally basic – the principle of respect for persons. Each person is a being of immeasurable value, a centre of rights and obligations, and may not be dealt with either as an object or as a commodity. Together, these two principles shape the nature and direction of our social ethics.

The health care field illustrates this in a series of assertions about the availability of health care services. These may perhaps best be summed up in the following claim: everyone, no matter who or where, how old, or what sex, condition, financial status, or religious persuasion, has an equal right to whatever techniques, resources, and treatment modalities that are available, for as long as he or she needs them. Anything less is a denial of equality and lack of respect.

Nor is this position merely a matter of common sentiment. It also finds expression at governmental levels. The Hall Report of 1964 first stated it officially (Royal Commission on Health Services in Canada 1964), the Lalonde Report of 1974 reiterated it as a matter of federal policy (Canadian Government Working Document 1974), and its thrust has recently been reaffirmed by federal pronouncements and actions on extra-billing.[1] Acceptance and institution of universal and comprehensive health care coverage at the various provincial levels amount to a similar endorsement, and although several provinces have toyed with the idea of extra-billing, not one of them has advanced the notion in order to deny the right to equal health care. Those who have considered it have done so because of an anticipated *in terrorem* effect which would curtail suspected abuses and/or overuses of the system. The aim, therefore, has been to lighten the economic burden that the idea of an equal right has placed on provincial coffers.

However – and my last remark provides the cue — the idea of equal, universal, and comprehensive access to health care (which is how the concept of an equal right is usually translated) neither is nor can be realized in practice. It assumes an unlimited amount of resources. This assumption is unrealistic in the best of times. Health care resources are finite. Nor is this limitation a political artifact. It stems from the nature of human society. All human societies are finite, which means that they can generate only a finite resource pool. Health care resources must be drawn from this pool, along with all others. Therefore, although the limits of the resources allocated to health care may be drawn differently compared to other areas of social endeavour, the fact of limitation itself will always remain.

Furthermore, any such redrawing of limits would have to occur with due regard for the legitimacy of other areas of social endeavour – education, social services, defence, and so on. Therefore it could not proceed arbitrarily, particularly since these other areas could also lay claim to the principles of equality and respect for persons as their foundation. It would have to take place within ethically mandated constraints that balanced the legitimacy of their competing claims. The best that could be hoped for would be an increase in the limits, never their removal; and while that increase might provide some relief from the immediate need for selective allocation within the health care field, sooner or later the new limits will also be reached and the need for selection will recur.

SOME DEMOGRAPHIC CONSIDERATIONS

This will be the case if our society is not static – and here the following considerations become relevant. Current analyses of Canadian demographic trends indicate that the chronological make-up of our society is undergoing a profound change. Assuming a low growth rate scenario, it is estimated that between the years 1981 and 2001, the number of people sixty-five years and older will rise from 2,360,900 to 3,884,500 – an increase of 64.5 per cent. With a total expected population of 28,529,200 by 2001, this means that approximately 13.6 per cent of the population will fall into that age bracket, compared to 9.7 per cent in 1981 (Statistics Canada 1985).

If life is a good and longevity a cause for rejoicing, then these figures should be welcomed. And yet, because resources are limited, these data are cause for concern. The same projections that we have just quoted also estimate that the dependency ratio of those sixty-five years and older – that is, the number of dependent people sixty-five years and older per 100 population (Statistics Canada 1985) – will rise from 15.6 to 24.4 within the same period, an increase of 56.4 per cent. It will reach 37.8 by the year 2021 and 51.6 by the year 2031 – an increase of 231 per cent over the 1981 figure (Statistics Canada 1985).

But even these figures do not tell the whole story. It is expected that while this monumental increase in dependents is taking place, the number of non-dependent and so-called "productive" persons – those between the ages of 18 and 64 – is expected to drop to 65.3 per cent of the population by 2001, to 62.8 per cent by 2021, and to 58.5 per cent by 2031 (Statistics Canada 1985). If we then take into account that an aging population increasingly consumes health care resources – proportionally the greatest consumption of health care resources occurs in the last years of life[2] – and the further fact that even with increased productivity, the amount of resources available to the health care sector is not expected to be nearly as great as the projected increase in the dependent elderly population, it becomes quite clear that these demographic changes will cause an acute allocation problem.

SOME CONTEMPORARY APPROACHES

How do we allocate resources in a selective and discriminatory fashion without violating the principles of equality and respect for persons? The problem is not, of course, entirely in the future. For some time now, health care decisionmakers have experienced the growing impact of the trends that we have sketched. Their responses have fallen – and continue to fall – into two categories. One is absolutistic in nature. It consists in focusing on the demographically identifiable group that is perceived to be responsible for the problem – the elderly – and attempting to solve the problem by dealing essentially with that group alone. More specifically, it centres on the contention that because it is this group and its disproportionately large drain on health care resources that is the cause of the rising resource insufficiency, the solution must consist in placing a bar on its access to health care. That bar, in turn, takes two forms. On the micro-level of individual allocation, it consists in a refusal to provide certain types of services that are available to all others – for example, by-pass surgery, dialysis, and organ transplants (President's Commission for the Study of Ethical Problems in Medicine and Biomedical and Behavioral Research 1983; Schwartz and Grubb 1985). On the macro-level of budgetary policy it manifests itself in the refusal to fund (or in an underfunding of) research into diseases and provision of health services that are typically appropriate for the aging.

The second, calculative type of approach is not quite so blatant or direct –

but it is just as effective. It consists in the adoption of allegedly neutral criteria of discriminatory (selective) allocation, their application to all relevant patient categories, and the decision to restrict treatment access to all and only those groups that meet them. These criteria are exemplified by cost-benefit and cost-effectiveness approaches (Feeny et al. 1986; Moskop 1987). It just so happens that the cost-benefit coefficients of many high-cost treatment modalities for the elderly are lower than those for other age groups, and that their cost-effectiveness coefficients are below what are considered to be reasonable levels. Transplantation, extensive orthopedic surgery, and neurosurgical interventions are implicated here. Consequently, in line with this approach, they are not generally made available in the geriatric setting (Schwartz and Grubb 1985).

By and large, the types of services that are withheld form the elderly are the same with either approach. Furthermore, both have been defended, if not in exactly the same way then at least by an appeal to the same principle: the principle of equality. The absolutistic approach has been defended by maintaining that the elderly "have already lived," that they have already had a chance at the various services and that it is now someone else's turn; and in any case, that equality is preserved because everyone who reaches the relevant age will be treated in the same fashion (President's Commission 1983). The calculative approach is defended by arguing that it is not inherently unethically discriminatory because all age groups have the same chance to meet the relevant criteria. It merely happens that the older age group is captured. It might have been any other. Equality is therefore preserved because all are subject to the same criteria and are treated in the same fashion.

ANALYSIS

Upon examination, however, neither of these approaches is ethically defensible. While the absolutistic one does not violate the principle of respect for persons, its preservation of equality is illusory. To begin with, it singles out those who are sixty-five and older as the only chronologically identifiable group that is subject to access restrictions. They, as a group, are said to cause the problem. If there were no such group, or if we ignored their special needs, the problem would disappear.

However, even if that were true, there is no a priori ethical reason why these considerations (assuming they were legitimate) should be applied only to this age group. They can also be applied, and with equal force, to other chronologically identifiable groups – for example, to neonates between zero and one years of age – who also have special and exceedingly cost-intensive needs. One look at the budgetary requirements of neonatal intensive care units will confirm this (Bennett & Feeny 1986). If equality were truly to be preserved and old age not to underlie this as a hidden agenda, then this group and others like it would have to be subjected to the same restrictive access rules based on the same reasoning. Very few of those who advocate the absolutistic approach are willing to see their reasoning applied in this fashion.

One could of course retreat to a secondary stance and argue that the two sorts of cases are entirely different: that the older age group has already had its chance at access to the disputed resources whereas the younger age groups have not, and that because of this the latter should have the first opportunity when it comes to allocation. Equality of opportunity demands it. This is what really lies behind the claim that the older age group "has already lived."

In a sense, and to a degree, this kind of reply can be defended, at least with respect to children. In their case – so one can argue – society has allowed new persons to come into existence knowing full well that they will be incompetent and dependent, and have needs that they cannot meet on their own. Consequently – so the reasoning may continue – by allowing them to develop to the point where they have become persons, the older, mature members of society have de facto subordinated their otherwise equal rights to those of the incompetent persons (Kluge 1975).

However, while admittedly defensible, this reply would not establish the intended thesis: it would not show that only those sixty-five years and older should have reduced access. Quite the contrary. It would show that all age groups over, say eighteen, would be in the same position because all, as competent adults, de facto would have subordinated their rights in a similar fashion. Refusal to act consistently on this conclusion would show the absolutistic approach for what it really is – a politically motivated violation of equality.

The approach also violates equality in another fashion. By its very nature, it affects only those over sixty-five years whose needs transcend the societal average. It would leave untouched all those who are blessed, if not with perfect health, then at least with a health status that is statistically average for society as a whole. It therefore effectively – and deliberately – discriminates only against those who have a greater than average need precisely because of the fact of that need. It would thereby reinforce any health status disadvantages that might exist in the group, and thereby magnify inequality. In no other context would we accept such a position. We would insist that individual differences have to be taken into account when trying to determine what is equitable and just; and we would insist that to aim a restrictive policy precisely at those who have a greater than average need is the rankest form of discrimination.

Finally, even if we were to ignore all this and the absolutistic approach were to be accepted, equality would demand consistency of application in practice. That would mean that no one – neither the Queen nor the Prime

Minister, neither the chief surgeon of a hospital, nor a genius like Albert Einstein, nor a humanitarian like Albert Schweitzer – may be exempted from this condition. The only way to avoid this conclusion would be to argue that exceptions are built into the absolutistic approach to cover such cases. However, in order to be ethically defensible these conditions may not be person-specific. They must involve criteria which, in principle, any person could meet. It is not at all clear, however, how such criteria could be defended except by reference to the necessity of such individuals for society's survival or in terms of reward for individual merit. As to society's survival, no one has as yet been able to show that only individuals from a certain age group must occupy a certain office or position in order for society to survive. In other words, this criterion again is not age-specific. As to individual merit, that criterion hides more of a program than a specific idea. In order for it to be useful, we would first have to clarify what sort of merit was involved, why it should be thought to be ethically relevant in this connection – and why we should assume that in fact the majority of the older age group would not possess it.

CALCULATIVE APPROACHES: COST-BENEFIT

If anything, the calculative approaches fare worse. To begin with cost-benefit considerations (Drummond 1986): in order to be meaningful, even on a merely theoretical level, they require that directly or indirectly persons must be treated as entities that have a numerical value, where that value can be expressed in terms equivalent to those of social goods and services. Otherwise no comparison to cost, and hence no evaluation, is possible.

The present context imposes severe limits on the depth of our argumentation, but at least four points should be raised. First, the very attempt to represent a person as equivalent to a calculable quantity violates the principle of respect for persons. That principle, let us recall, characterizes persons as entities of immeasurable value and as centres of rights and obligations. In short, it characterizes them not as quantifiable objects or commodities but as entities without price. The very attempt at cost-benefit calculation, therefore, must be rejected as involving a violation of one of our most fundamental ethical beliefs (Kluge 1986).

This aside, however, whatever discriminatory power cost-benefit analysis has for the present context derives from its inconsistent application. After all, when it is applied consistently it is not age-specific. Rather, it picks out all and only those cases where the relevant cost-benefit quotient is not present. That, however, means that it will not pick out everyone who is sixty-five or over; only those in whose case the quotient is not present. At the same time it will pick out some who are younger than sixty-five, and for the same reason.

It will therefore also pick out some who are younger but congenitally defective, severely retarded, crippled, or otherwise severely handicapped. Once more, it is not at all clear that proponents of this approach would accept such a consequence. Not to accept it, however, while insisting on it in the case of the aged, is to violate the principle of equality.

Furthermore, the cost-benefit approach is difficult to defend from a pragmatic perspective. It requires that a specific value be assigned to the benefits expected. While that may, just barely, be possible for middle-aged and older persons, it is virtually impossible to do so for those eighteen and younger without begging the question. In their case we lack sufficient data to be able to project with anything like precision. Also, whatever the projections of evaluation and benefit we make, in order to be calculatively useful they depend on assuming an accurate view of social change – something no one has as yet been able to produce.

Finally, cost-benefit analysis is workable if and only if there has been some previous identification – and defence – of the quantitative limits of expected benefits, and indeed of their very nature. That, however, takes us squarely into the debate between those who see the function of health care to be caring and those who see it as curing; between those who promote a prevention-oriented health care approach and those who have a crisis orientation. It also takes us into the debate over what constitutes genuine and defensible values in the human context. None of these issues are even close to being resolved. Without a resolution, however, cost-benefit analysis is reduced to a mere shibboleth to rally support for what is an arbitrarily decided matter of expediency (Drummond 1986).

COST-EFFECTIVENESS

Cost-effectiveness considerations, of course, escape these criticisms. Superficially at least, they avoid confronting the principle of respect for persons because they do not require us to equate persons with some calculable value, directly or otherwise. They focus solely on the relative effectiveness of the relevant procedures vis-à-vis their cost; and by insisting on the same cost-effectiveness coefficients for all, they appear to guarantee equality.

Nevertheless, cost-effectiveness analysis also faces certain problems. Like cost-benefit analysis, it is not inherently age-specific. Therefore it will capture neither all who are sixty-five or over nor only those. It will also capture sufferers from AIDS, MS, and MD, radically defective neonates, and those who have Parkinson's or Alzheimer's diseases – to mention but a few examples. The only way to avoid the inclusion of these people is once more to return to arbitrary decision making – and thereby abandon all pretense at ethical concern.

Second, the criterion itself is not ethically neutral. The effectiveness of a particular treatment modality for a given context is functionally dependent on the level of medico-technological, pharmacological, and surgical sophistication that obtains in the relevant area. This is but to say that it is functionally determined by the amount of money society is willing to commit to that area in terms of research and development (R and D). The commitment of R and D funds, however, is a political matter centering on what priorities are deemed important. To that extent, therefore, an appeal to cost-effectiveness considerations as a reason for curtailing certain services to the elderly is nothing more than a covert attempt at legitimizing a preconceived value scheme. (It will also be apparent that unless that value scheme is challenged, health care which does not currently meet cost-effectiveness requirements will be caught in a vicious circle: failure to meet the requirements leads to failure to fund, which leads to failure to develop, which leads to failure to meet cost-effectiveness requirements, which leads to –).

Third, while it may be clear what is meant by "cost" in cost-effectiveness considerations – although even that clarity may be illusory[3] – the concept of effectiveness is inherently and systematically ambiguous. The effectiveness of a procedure is not an absolute matter contained in the nature of the procedure itself. It is relative to the reason why the procedure is employed. For instance, a colon resection may be performed to improve the quality of life of a given individual, to save his life, or simply as an expression of deep and enduring concern and care (Ramsey 1970). In each of these cases, the effectiveness may be evaluated differently, although the nature and cost of the procedure remains the same. A mere comparison of cost-effectiveness coefficients will not capture that difference, and hence will be logically skewed – like comparing apples with ants. The point may be put generally. Cost-effectiveness considerations, by separating the functioning of a particular modality in a material sense from the reason for its employment, commits the fallacy of isolation. A realistic assessment demands that the context inclusive of the end aimed at and the values pursued form the framework within which the effectiveness of a procedure is determined. Since these may vary not merely from age group to age group (Gutman et al. 1986) but even from case to case within a specific age group, cost-effectiveness considerations have at best a very narrow window of employment (Drummond 1986). Certainly, to base a policy of selective allocation directed explicitly against gerontologically-oriented health care on them would be entirely unwarranted.

EQUALITY

So far my remarks have been entirely negative, and while they may be useful in pointing out that certain well-established approaches amount to ethical dead ends, this does not really advance the issue. The need for allocation – for selective and discriminatory allocation – remains as real as it is pressing. At the same time, we are unwilling to give up our ethical beliefs. Is there a way to reconcile the two and resolve the issue?

Perhaps we can make a start by re-examining the concept of equality. Equality does not mean sameness. That point may be illustrated in the following way. In an egalitarian society of materially identical beings, there are no differences in the health care needs of different persons. Since all are materially identical and subject to the same conditions, their needs are the same. By way of analogy, the situation could be compared to the relationship that holds among points on the surface of a sphere: their curvature relationship is the same.

Reality, however, is different. The material nature, social positions, and health care needs of people differ. To continue the analogy, this difference can be likened to the distortions of the surface of the sphere as a result of variations in the stress of the metric which connects the points. However – and here we come to the point of the analogy – we can develop mathematical functions that allow us to treat the various points in a *qualitatively* identical fashion despite the *quantitative* differences of the surface metric in which they are embedded. These are called topological functions. They preserve qualitative identity despite quantitative difference. The requirement of equality that we are trying to achieve – of treating individuals qualitatively the same as persons despite their quantitative differences as material beings – is like this. In this sense, equality is a topological relation. And just as geometric topological relations require that we treat different points quantitatively differently precisely in order to preserve their qualitative identity, so ethical ones require that we treat materially different persons in a quantitatively distinctive fashion in order to ensure their qualitative equality. In more concrete terms, it means that the principle of equality requires not sameness of allocation but difference: a difference that is functionally determined by the differences in the health status of the relevant persons.[4]

Can this be applied to the problem that faces us? Let us go back to the claim that everyone has an equal right to health care. What precisely does the notion of health care amount to? A useful way of interpreting it is in terms of acts directed toward individuals. On that understanding, it would be reasonable to suppose that an equal right to health care is a right to equal treatment in the delivery of such acts. Of course, health care acts differ in nature, complexity, and so on. In each case, however, we can establish a correlation between the intended and the actual outcome of the act, irrespective of cost. That correlation can be expressed as a coefficient: the act-effectiveness coefficient. We can then say that the right to equal health care is the right not to be disadvantaged in the degree of care one receives in the delivery of health care services relative to other persons; and this, in turn, can now be expressed quantitatively by saying that the act-effectiveness coefficient of the relevant health care acts for all people must be essentially the same.

THE CALCULUS OF DISCRIMINATION

All of this has to be worked into an allocation policy that recognizes the fact of resource limitation; and if, as we have assumed all along, the principle of respect for persons is fundamental to our ethical outlook, then we must begin with micro-allocation (which is directed towards the individual) rather than macro-allocation (which is directed towards groups).

The basic and absolute condition of equality may be expressed like this:

(1) Everyone has a right to the same basic measure of health care resources as everyone else, where the level and nature of these is functionally determined by the average health status profile for members of that society, its socio-economic capabilities, medical sophistication, and competing areas of legitimate social concern.[5]

It is clear from this that any a priori exclusion of the elderly from available health care resources that are standard measure, solely by virtue of age, is indefensible.

If we call (1) primacy allocation, then we can formulate a condition of secondary allocation to reflect differential needs:

(2) If the health status of an individual is lower than the statistical norm for that society, then a secondary allocation is prima facie mandated.

Clause (2) is an attempt to preserve equality in the face of quantitative material difference. Like (1), it entails that failure to provide needed services – for example, heart transplant, hip replacement, by-pass surgery, or even dialysis – to an elderly person solely because of age is clearly unethical because it seems to violate equality.

However, (2) merely sets the stage. Lower-than-average health status may not be the result of heteronomous factors beyond the individual's control but may be auto-induced, for example, the result of knowingly persisting in alcohol abuse, imprudent life style, and so on. Alternatively, it may be hetero-induced but the attempt to correct the situation may require a degree of care that transcends what equality dictates. Therefore, to preserve justice and avoid reverse discrimination, the following conditions must also be met:

(3) A prima facie right to secondary allocation becomes actual if and only if (a) the lower-than-average status is not auto-induced[6] and (b) the act-effectiveness coefficient of procedures contemplated under (2) falls within the range of coefficients for procedures mandated under (1).

With this we have the first reasons for selective allocation. Not, however, on the basis of age but on the basis of the origin of the relevant needs and of the requirements for meeting them. These conditions apply to all persons.

We now have to address the fact of resource limitation directly. This can be done by the following clauses:

(4) All secondary allocation claims must be ranked according to nature. Those that involve saving/preserving life take priority over those that preserve/improve quality; and those that are need-driven (that is, where the condition will deteriorate irreparably with time) take priority over those that are not.

(5) If the health status of the disadvantaged person under (3), after secondary allocation, is not equal to or better than it was before (where this is traceable to the fact of secondary allocation itself) then the obligation to provide secondary allocation ceases.

The reason for (4) centres on the priority ranking of the right to health care. I have discussed the matter elsewhere (Kluge 1986) and therefore shall leave it at that. As to (5), its reason lies in the concept of health care itself. Providing health care is not like servicing a car. There, a modular approach is possible; we need not take the functioning of the car as a whole into account. In health care the focus is on health: the state of homeostatic balance of the organism as a whole that allows it to fulfill its genetically determined function (Dubos 1959).[7] From that perspective, health care directed towards maintaining/improving the functioning of a particular organ, system, or subsystem without regard to overall health status is misdirected. In order to be mandated by the right to *health* care, the overall health status must be implicated. This of course means that (5) may bar an elderly person from access to certain treatment modalities. For example, it would bar a sixty-eight-year-old brittle diabetic in chronic and progressive renal failure with severe vascular and eye involvement from being a candidate for by-pass surgery. However, it would not bar access for a seventy-two-year-old in otherwise acceptable health and with good prognosis for recovery.

Equality mandates positive secondary allocation. However, it also mandates limitation if the result of that allocation amounts to reverse discrimination. This may be expressed as follows:

(6) The health status of the initially disadvantaged person as a result of the secondary allocation must not be higher than that of the average health status under (1).

MACRO-ALLOCATION

The above sketch presents a scheme for ethically acceptable discriminatory resource allocation at the micro-level under conditions of limitation. While it does not focus on age, it will capture some of the aged. Not, however, because they are elderly, but because, along with some others, they do not meet the conditions that everyone else must meet.

This scheme can be transformed into a macro-allocation scheme by a statistical analysis of the actual and projected distribution pattern mandated by clauses (1) to (6) (Kluge 1986). That, in turn, will point the way to formulating budgetary policies. These policies may not be age-focused – indeed, will not be – and therefore will not be directed against the elderly per se. They will be health care allocation policies that apply equally to all persons, and that allow for an identification of groups only insofar as that is medically necessary.

This denouement may be perceived as failing to address the problem of allocation brought on by the increase in the number of the aged. To argue this, however, is to insist on what we have exposed as a fallacy: the claim that, by definition, the problem must be solved by remaining within the traditional framework that sees age as decisive. We must always keep in mind that if the problem is how to allocate limited health care resources in an ethically acceptable fashion, without violating personhood and equality, then these principles must be the guiding parameters for any solution, not some preconceived idea of what the solution must look like. What we have sketched meets that requirement. At the same time, it is discriminatory and will put limits on how much of the resources any group of individuals may consume. These limits will exist not because of any a priori assumption about what the limits must be for the group as a whole, but because of the internal limits that the micro-allocation formulae place on individual consumption within the group.

CONCLUSION

If what we have argued is correct, then although the scarcity of health care resources may be exacerbated by the demographic shift towards greater age, it would be unethical to try to solve the allocation problem by discriminating against the elderly. It is also programmatically unnecessary to do so. The allocation criteria that we have sketched allow for an equitable resource distribution that respects the personhood of each individual while being sensitive to the facts of limited resources and differential needs. We may accept as a truism that the number of health care problems increases with age, and that the demographic trend indicated will have its material effects on our society's ability to provide care. However, to operate as though these facts mandated distinctive treatment is to confuse the enabling condition for the problem with the problem itself. No one ceases to be a person because he becomes older, nor does old age strip him of his right to equality. Discrimination is acceptable if it occurs on the basis of ethically relevant differences; otherwise, it is unjust.

What we have sketched is merely a beginning, not a complete solution. Several problems remain unaddressed. Most crucial perhaps is the issue of how to determine the level of primary allocation. Our suspicion is that it can be resolved by considering the types of health care problems that are usually encountered by members of our society under the prevailing socio-economic, environmental, and other conditions, and by a judicious balancing of the health of our society's members against other social goods. This last, however, is not merely a matter of rights. It also involves values – and thereby transcends the limits of the present discussion.

NOTES

1 The basis of this is discussed in Justice Emmett Hall (1980).
2 Estimates here vary. However, Gutman et al. (1986) suggest that purely from the standpoint of hospitalization, those 70 years and older use hospital services on a bed-per-capita basis 2 ½ to 5 times more than those between 55 and 60. Likewise, the average fee-for-service cost per person per year rises from $400 between 0 and 64 to $815.50 per male per year and $537.90 per female per year between 65 and 85 (Gutman et al. 1986).
3 Despite attempts by some researchers – for example, Torrance (1982) and Wolfson et al. (1982) – it is not at all clear how parameters like psychological trauma, social disruption, personal affect, and so on can be expressed in fiscal terms.
4 We here assume that the differences are not auto-induced.
5 This is similar to Fried (1976). For a different approach see Daniels (1985) and President's Commission (1983). The latter contains a whole series of noteworthy discussions on resource allocation in vol. 2.
6 Clearly, this requires further discussion. See also Bayer (1981).
7 For other analyses of health, see Callahan (1973), Englehardt (1981), Feinberg (1974).

REFERENCES

Bayer, R. (1981). Voluntary health risks and public policy. *Hastings Center Report,* 11(5), 26

Bennett, K., & Feeny, D. (1986). Clinical and economic evaluation of therapeutic technologies: The case of neonatal intensive care programs. In Feeney et al. (Eds.), *Health care technology: Effectiveness, efficiency and public policy.* Montreal: Institute for Research on Public Policy

Callahan, D. (1973). The WHO definition of health. *Hastings Center Studies.* 1(3), 77–87

Daniels, N. (1985). *Just health care.* Cambridge: Cambridge University Press

Drummond, M. (1986). Guidelines for health technology assessment: Economic evaluation. In Feeny et al. (Eds.), *Health care technology: effectiveness, efficiency and public policy.* Montreal: Institute for Research on Public Policy

Dubos, R. (1959). *Mirage of health.* New York: Harper & Row

Englehardt, H.T., Jr. (1981). Human well-being and medicine: Some basic value--judgments in the biological sciences. In T.H. Mappes and J.S. Zembaty (Eds.), *Biomedical ethics*. New York: McGraw-Hill

Feeny, D., Guyatt, G., & Tugwell, P. (Eds.). (1986). *Health care technology: Effectiveness, efficiency and public policy*. Montreal: Institute for Research on Public Policy

Feinberg, J. (1974). Disease and value. In *Doing and deserving: Essays in the theory of responsibility*. Princeton, NJ: Princeton University Press

Fried, C. (1976). Equality and rights in medical care. *Hastings Center Report*. 6(1), 29–34

Gutman, G.M., Gee, E.U., Bojanowski, B.C., & Mottet, D. (1986). *Fact book on aging in British Columbia*. Burnaby, B.C.: Simon Fraser University Gerontology Research Centre

Hall, Justice E. (1980). *Canada's national provincial health program for the 1980s: A commitment for renewal*. Ottawa: Department of National Health and Welfare

Kluge, E.W. (1975). *The practice of death*. New Haven: Yale University Press

———. (1986). Once and future persons: Ethical reflections on health care delivery for the elderly in the year 2000. In *Health care for the elderly for the year 2000*. Symposium Proceedings, B.C. Ministry of Health (November 1987)

Lalonde, M. (1974). *A new perspective on the health of Canadians: A working document* (Lalonde Report). Ottawa: Department of National Health and Welfare Canada

Moskop, J.C. (1987). The moral limits to federal funding for kidney disease. *Hastings Center Report*, 17(2), 11–15

President's Commission for the Study of Ethical Problems in Medicine and Biomedical and Behavioral Research. (1983). Securing access to health care, 3 vols. Washington, DC: U.S. Government Printing Office

Ramsey, P. (1970). *The patient as person*. New Haven: Yale University Press

Royal Commission on Health Services in Canada, vol. 1 (1964). Justice Emmett Hall, Chairman (Hall Report) Ottawa: Queen's Printer

Schwartz, R., & Grubb, A. (1985). Why Britain can't afford informed consent. *Hastings Center Report,* 15(4), 19–25

Statistics Canada (1985). *Population projections for Canada, provinces and territories: 1984–2006. Catalogue 91–510*. Ottawa: Statistics Canada

Torrance, G.W. (1982). Preferences for health states: A review of measurement methods. In J.C. Sinclair (Ed.), *Clinical and economic evaluation of perinatal program*. Mead Johnson Symposium on Perinatal and Developmental Medicine, Colorado

Wolfson, A.D., Sinclair, A.J., Bombardier, C., & McGeer, A. (1982). Preference measurements for functional states in stroke patients: Interrater and intertechnique comparisons. In R.L. Kane and R.A. Kane (Eds.), *Values and long-term care*. Lexington, MA: D.C. Heath

8

Population Aging and the Economy: Some Issues in Resource Allocation

FRANK T. DENTON AND BYRON G. SPENCER

INTRODUCTION

A *stationary* population is one that is constant in both size and composition.[1] Individuals age and eventually die but they are replaced by identical individuals. Births and immigration are equal to deaths and emigration. As each cohort moves up the age ladder it is replaced by a younger cohort of the same size and characteristics. The numerical relations among age groups thus do not change: there is a fixed number of children for every adult, a fixed number of old people per person of working age; there are no changes in the proportions of families with school-age children, of old age pensioners, of workers, of young voters and old voters. Once the distribution of societal resources or income has been established – through economic, political, and social processes – there are no demographic influences to alter that distribution.

A population that is in *steady-state growth* is increasing at a constant rate, but again its age distribution is unchanging in relative terms. Every age group grows at the same constant rate and the different groups in the population again remain in fixed ratios to one another. One can conceive of society as determining how its total resources will be allocated among age groups in this case too, and, once determined, the allocation rule would require no revision for demographic reasons.

The concepts of a stationary population and steady-state growth are useful for demographic analysis but are not ones with which any real human population is ever likely to conform. Birth rates change, for biological, sociological, or economic reasons that may be only vaguely understood, and are not predictable with any degree of confidence in the present state of knowledge. Death rates decline, as a result of improvements in nutrition, health care technology or availability, and so on, or they rise, as a result of wars, famine, and epidemics. Patterns of migration shift for political or socio-economic reasons, both nationally and internationally. All such changes have implications for the age distribution of the population. They create social and political tensions and may result in a collective reconsideration of the rules and criteria for allocating the national output among groups at different stages of the life course.

We are going through such a process of reconsideration in Canada. The same is true of the United States and other nations. The "baby bust" of the 1960s and 1970s, following hard on the heels of the "baby boom" of the 1940s and 1950s, has created an unprecedented shift in the age structure of the Canadian population and the prospect of further major shifts in the next few decades – and indeed beyond, for changes in birth rates have repercussions which persist very far into the future.

The three most obvious areas of resource use affected by changes in age structure are education, pensions, and health care. The concern about "population aging" usually focuses on the prospective "burden" of future support for a greatly enlarged population of old people, including the higher levels of hospital, medical, and related costs that such an elderly population will require. At the same time, the sharply reduced proportion of children has reduced the need for expenditures on schools and universities, and unless there is a marked (and unanticipated) rise in the birth rate, this will continue to serve at least as a potential offset to higher old-age-related costs. (Educational costs, like those of other services, obviously do not depend only on demographic factors; however, it is these with which we are concerned here.)

But the economic effects of population change are much broader than this. Population change affects not only the demands for age-related services but the ability of the economy to provide them and, more generally, to produce the whole range of services and commodities that we refer to as the gross national product. To consider only the demand effects of population aging is to miss half the picture; supply effects must be considered also to get things into proper perspective.

Questions of who gets what – of how the national product is to be shared when resources are limited (as they always are) – obviously have large ethical content. We are not concerned in this paper with ethical issues themselves but rather with providing some background against which the issues can be identified and assessed more clearly. Our aim is an objective discussion and analysis of the population aging process and its likely effects on various aspects of the Canadian economy in the decades ahead.

The paper proceeds as follows: the next section offers a review of changes in the Canadian population and associated changes in the labour force, and then a look into the (always murky) future. "How Does Population Change Affect the Economy?" provides a general discussion of these effects and the adjustment problems that result. Some aspects of intergenerational relations are examined in "The Arithmetic of Integenerational Dependency" by the use of alternative calculations of past and future "dependency ratios" within the Canadian population. A model of an economic-demographic system is introduced in the next section, as a vehicle for simulating simultaneously the supply and demand effects of population change at the level of the macroeconomy. The effects of future population change on government budgets in Canada are then considered. In succeeding sections, further attention is directed to the three most age-sensitive components of public expenditure, namely, pensions, health care, and education, making use again of the economic-demographic simulation model. This is followed by some concluding remarks.

THE CANADIAN POPULATION AND LABOUR FORCE: PAST, PRESENT, AND FUTURE

We have made a series of projections of the Canadian population and labour force to the year 2051. Three of our projection sets are shown in Table 1, together with historical figures back to 1921. The table shows population totals, annual growth rates by decade, and distributions by age. It shows also the corresponding labour force totals and growth rates.

The projections that we have made are based on alternative assumptions about fertility, mortality, and migration rates.[2] The three that we have chosen to display in Table 1 are what we term our "standard" projection and projections based on "high" and "low" fertility rates. Somewhat surprisingly, perhaps, the economic effects of population aging depend much more critically on what happens to the birth rate than on changes in mortality rates. The effects of alternative migration levels are also much less important than birth rate effects.

Let us begin by reviewing the history of population change. The population of Canada was recorded as about 8.8 million at the 1921 census; by the 1981 census it had reached about 24.3 million. In between there was a series of profound demographic changes.

The birth rate fell during the 1920s and most of the 1930s, and immigration was down sharply from the levels of earlier in the century. Accordingly, the rates of population growth fell too. The growth rate was 2.0 per cent per annum in the decade ending in 1921 but only 1.0 in the decade ending in 1941. The proportion of children also fell and the proportion of older people rose: 12.1 per cent of the population were under five years of age in 1921,

TABLE 1: The Population and Labour Force of Canada:
Historical 1921–81; Projected 1991–2051

	Population						Labour force	
Year	Total ("000)	Annual growth rate(%)	Distribution by age (%) 0–4	5–19	20–64	65+	Total ("000)	Annual growth rate(%)
1921	8,788	2.0	12.1	31.5	51.6	4.8	3,284	1.7
1931	10,377	1.7	10.4	31.3	52.8	5.6	4,013	2.0
1941	11,507	1.0	9.1	28.4	55.8	6.7	4,612	1.4
1951	14,009	2.0	12.3	25.7	54.4	7.8	5,205	1.2
1961	18,238	2.7	12.4	29.5	50.6	7.6	6,631	2.5
1971	21,568	1.9	8.4	31.0	52.5	8.1	8,737	2.8
1981	24,342	1.2	7.3	24.7	58.3	9.7	12,158	3.3
			Standard					
1991	27,055	1.1	7.2	20.6	60.9	11.3	14,311	1.6
2001	29,120	.7	5.9	20.1	61.6	12.4	15,975	1.1
2011	30,620	.5	5.6	17.7	62.9	13.7	16,695	.4
2021	31,696	.3	5.4	16.8	60.2	17.6	16,359	—.2
2031	32,025	.1	5.1	16.5	56.7	21.8	15,871	–.3
2041	31,689	–.1	5.1	15.9	56.8	22.1	15,651	–.1
2051	30,987	–.2	5.1	16.1	56.8	22.0	15,263	–.3
			High Fertility					
1991	28,416	1.6	10.6	20.8	57.8	10.7	14,281	1.6
2001	33,091	1.5	9.1	26.0	54.1	10.8	16,096	1.2
2011	37,622	1.3	9.2	24.8	54.9	11.2	18,577	1.4
2021	43,821	1.5	10.3	24.4	52.5	12.7	20,538	1.0
2031	50,200	1.4	9.5	26.7	49.9	13.9	23,181	1.2
2041	57,411	1.4	10.1	25.6	52.1	12.2	27,508	1.7
2051	66,317	1.5	10.2	26.4	52.7	10.7	31,645	1.4
			Low Fertility					
1991	26,812	1.0	6.6	20.6	61.5	11.4	14,317	1.6
2001	28,411	.6	5.3	18.8	63.2	12.7	15,954	1.1
2011	29,417	.3	5.0	16.0	64.7	14.3	16,359	.3
2021	29,813	.1	4.6	15.1	61.7	18.7	15.615	–.5
2031	29,401	–.1	4.2	14.4	57.7	23.7	14.654	–.6
2041	28,270	–.4	4.2	13.8	57.2	24.8	13,860	–.6
2051	26,715	–.6	4.2	13.9	56.6	25.3	13,000	–.6

Growth rates refer to the decade preceding each of the indicated years.

9.1 per cent in 1941; 4.8 per cent of the population were sixty-five or older in 1921, 6.7 per cent in 1941.

The situation turned around sharply in the 1940s. Fertility rates rose to levels that were completely unanticipated and that would have seemed incredible only a few years earlier. The baby boom was under way and it was to last until the beginning of the 1960s. Population growth accelerated, reaching an annual rate of 2.7 per cent in the intercensal period 1951–61. The proportion of children rose sharply and the long-term trend toward higher proportions of older people was arrested. The effects on the school system were felt within the first few years, and persisted for a long time as the baby boom cohorts made their way through the elementary and secondary schools, and then on to the universities and colleges. The effects on the labour force came almost two decades later, but they were just as dramatic. The rapid economic expansion of the 1950s created a heavy demand for labour, but with the domestic supply not yet responding to the newly attained high levels of births, this demand had to be satisfied from foreign sources. It has been estimated that about half the increase in the Canadian labour force in the period 1951–61 is attributable to the high levels of net immigration.

The young "baby boomers" started to come into the labour market in the early and mid-1960s. The numbers of young workers began to grow rapidly and this growth continued right through the 1970s. By then the baby boom had already ended. Fertility rates began to slide noticeably in the early 1960s and the slide continued. The "baby bust" had commenced. Fertility rates continued to fall through the 1960s and the 1970s, reaching levels that were both unanticipated and without precedent in Canada. The total fertility rate – the average number of children that a woman would bear over the whole of her childbearing period – has fallen to 1.7 in recent years, well below the level of 2.1 necessary for the population just to replace itself in the long run.

The corresponding decreases in the proportions of children in the population have been very sharp: from 12.4 per cent in 1961, the proportion of children under five years of age had fallen to 7.3 per cent by 1981, with clear and important implications for the rate of labour-force growth in the decades ahead. At the same time, the long-run rise in the proportion of old people has resumed. As Table 1 shows, the proportion of people sixty-five or older exceeded the proportion of children under five in 1981 for the first time in the sixty-year history recorded in the table and, in all probability, for the first time in all of Canadian demographic history since the early days of European settlement. The phenomenon of population aging has been firmly re-established, bringing with it a host of concerns – well founded or otherwise – about its social and economic effects.

Our standard population projection assumes that the total fertility rate will remain at 1.7 children per woman, that mortality rates will continue to decline until 2026, but at a decelerating pace, and that net immigration will be 80,000 per annum (120,000 in, 40,000 out). The other two projections reported in Table 1 make the same assumptions about mortality and migration but different ones about fertility: the high fertility projection has the total fertility rate rising to 3.0 children per woman by 1991 and then remaining at that level; the low fertility one has the rate falling to 1.5 by 1991. The labour force projections assume in all cases a continuation of historical trends in participation rates (increases in the participation of women, further declines in the rates for the older population as the average age of retirement falls).

The population continues to rise for roughly the next four decades even under the low fertility assumption. (Under the high assumption it grows indefinitely.) However, the rate of growth falls off sharply under the standard and low assumptions. The proportion of children under five continues to decline under the standard and low assumptions, but rises sharply under the high assumption, as one would expect, since a total fertility rate of 3.0 implies a very large increase in the birth rate. The proportion of people sixty-five and older continues to rise sharply under the standard and low assumptions, and even under the high assumption there are substantial increases until the fourth decade of the next century. Measured in this way, the population aging process can be expected to continue for a long time, regardless of what happens to the birth rate. (A more rapid decline of mortality rates than we have assumed would increase the proportion of older people further, although the effects of mortality changes are generally much less pronounced than the effects of changes in fertility.) Under the standard assumptions, the population sixty-five or over rises from 9.7 per cent of the total population in 1981 to 12.4 per cent by 2001 and then to 22.0 by 2051. Although there are increases in every decade, the largest increases are still some decades away.

The projected patterns of labour force growth reflect the growth of the population and also its changing age distribution. From 3.3 per cent per annum in the decade 1971–81, the rate falls to 1.6 per cent in 1981–91 under all three sets of projection assumptions, and then to 1.1 or 1.2 per cent in the decade 1991–2001. Thereafter the labour force ceases to grow and then declines, in the standard and low projections; it continues to grow in the high projection but at much lower rates than we have experienced in Canada since the 1950s.

To summarize the outlook: (1) the population will continue to "age" for the next half-century, and very sharply unless there is a marked reversal of the trend in fertility rates; (2) population growth will continue until well into the next century, even with very low fertility rates, but the growth rate will be low and declining; (3) labour force growth will continue into the first two decades of the next century, but will then give way to declines unless fertility rates have risen by that time; and (4) further declines in the proportion of children can be expected over the next fifty years, in the absence of substantial fertility increases.

HOW DOES POPULATION CHANGE AFFECT THE ECONOMY?

Concerns about population aging usually focus on the implications for public expenditures, in particular, expenditures on health care and pensions. But the

TABLE 2: Major Economic Effects of Population Change and Associated Adjustment Problems

Supply Effects

Labour force – size, growth rate, and age composition affected; major impact of birth rate delayed 1½ to 2 decades but may be some immediate effect on female participation rates; mortality changes have negligible effect; immigration has immediate and direct effect

Productivity – effects related to age composition of labour force; young labour force less experienced on the one hand, but more recently trained and educated on the other

Capital stock – affected by rate of capital investment, which may be subject to demographic influences (see demand effects)

Potential GNP – economy's productive capacity affected by all of the above

Demand Effects

Private consumption – levels and patterns influenced by size and age composition of population and related rates of household formation and dissolution

Capital investment – affected by age-related changes in consumption demand

Public services – effects on public pensions, health care, education, and other budget categories as size and age composition of population changes

Exports – affected by population changes abroad (which may be similar to those in the exporting country if there are common demographic trends)

Adjustment Problems

Labour force – surpluses of some skills, shortages of others may develop as demand patterns change: How fast can the labour force adjust through inflows of young workers, outflows of older ones, training or retraining, migration, etc.? Can increased inflows of young workers, immigrants, or others be absorbed rapidly enough to avoid high rates of unemployment?

Capital stock – Surpluses or shortages of particular types of capital equipment and structures may develop as demand patterns change: How fast can the capital stock adjust through processes of depreciation, scrappage, new investment, and conversion of old stock to new uses?

Technological change – Does technological change worsen or ameliorate difficulties of adjustment in the labour force and the capital stock? Is the rate of technological change increased or decreased as a result of demographic change?

Industrial structure – Related to the above: How fast can the industrial structure of the economy shift in response to demographically induced changes in demand patterns? How fast can the geographic distribution of industry respond to population redistribution (and vice versa)?

Social and political – How fast, and to what extent, will society and elected governments respond to altered patterns of demand for public services and associated requirements for budgetary reallocations, tax changes, and changes in intergovernmental revenue sharing?

economic consequences of population aging – and of population change in general – are much broader than this. Indeed, virtually every aspect of the economy is affected, either directly or indirectly. A brief summary of the major effects is provided in Table 2 and the discussion in this section is centred on that table.

The effects can be classified as either supply or demand effects. On the supply side, the most obvious effect is on the labour force. For example, an increase in fertility levels engenders an increase in the supply of young workers some one and a half to two decades later. An increase in immigration has an immediate effect, since a large proportion of immigrants typically are of working age. But there are delayed effects also, as the children of immigrants become adults and enter the labour force – and then *their* children. Changes in mortality rates can have some effects on the labour force also, although these are generally of very small order. In the Canadian context, the level of fertility is likely to remain the most important demographic factor in determining the future course of labour force growth.

Changes in fertility affect the future age distribution of the labour force, and this has implications for the level of productivity. An increase in the proportion of young workers has two effects which pull in opposite directions. On the one hand, young workers are inexperienced ones. On the other hand, they are more recently trained and educated. To the extent that new technology requires new skills, the rate of entrance of young people into the work force may be a major consideration from the point of view of the economy's ability to implement new methods of production. The introduction or extension of computer training in the educational system from the elementary schools on is an obvious case in point.

The nation's capital stock is affected also by population change. The stock of equipment and structures is influenced by the rate of investment, and this in turn is subject to demographic influence, as we discuss below. Not only the size of the stock can be affected, but also its age structure and technological modernity: just as young workers are more likely to have modern skills, recently created physical capital may also reflect the newest techniques of production. Conversely, a older capital stock may be a less productive one.

The potential gross national product – the economy's *capacity* for production – is affected by all of these factors: changes in the size of the labour force, age-related changes in average productivity levels, and demographically induced changes in the size and composition of the capital stock.

Turning to the demand side of the economy, there are obvious effects on the levels and patterns of private consumption. For one thing, a larger population means "more mouths to feed," so to speak – or more literally, greater demands for food, shelter, clothing, transportation services, entertainment, and so on. But the age distribution of the population also matters, for patterns of consumption are different at different stages of the life cycle and rates of formation of new households and dissolution of old ones clearly are related to the proportions of young and old people in the population.

The demand for capital investment is related both directly and indirectly to the population, its rate of growth, and its age distribution. The demand for investment in new housing is obviously related very directly. The demand for investment in factories and machinery, on the other hand, may be influenced indirectly as a result of demographically induced changes in the demand for consumer goods.

The demand for public services is of particular concern in popular discussions of the problems of an aging population. Visions of huge armies of pensioners and massive requirements for hospital beds, nursing home facilities, and the like are conjured up. Not so often remembered in such discussions are the concomitant reductions in the size of the school-age population and the other effects that changes in the age distribution of the population can have on government budgets and revenue requirements. Even less frequently recognized are the supply effects noted above and their implications for the tax base from which government revenues are drawn.

Some of the population effects on consumption and investment manifest themselves as changes in demand for domestic goods and some as changes in demand for foreign goods. Thus the level and composition of imports may be affected. Moreover, demographic trends typically show little concern for national boundaries, and population changes abroad may result in changes in the demand for exports. This is particularly true of Canada: the low Canadian fertility rates are essentially a reflection of a North American phenomenon – indeed a phenomenon characteristic of much of the industrialized world. The demand for both Canadian exports and Canadian imports may thus be subject to influences arising from similar demographic sources.

We have referred to the effects of population changes on the potential gross national product. However, whether the economy reaches its potential depends on the rate at which it is able to adjust to shifts in demand patterns and changes in technology. There are thus important problems – or potential problems – of adjustment which must be taken into account.

Population change may induce changes in demands for goods, which imply altered demands for labour. Some skills may become surplus while others are in short supply. How fast the labour force can adjust may depend on how rapidly it is being augmented by influxes of young (recently trained) workers or immigrants, how rapidly it is being diminished by the retirement of older workers, the extent of training or retraining of the existing labour force, and so on. At the same time, if the influx of new workers is very rapid (as it was in the 1970s and early 1980s), the labour market may be unable to respond quickly enough. Thus, high levels of unemployment may result from limitations on the economy's capacity for absorbing new workers.

Surpluses or shortages of particular types of capital equipment and structures may result also from demographically induced shifts in demand. The question here is how fast the economy can adjust its capital stock through the processes of depreciation and scrappage on the one hand, and new investment and conversion of old stock to new uses on the other.

Technology does not stand still while population changes run their course and developments of technology may either complicate or assist the economy's adjustment processes. Technological change may increase the redundancy of some skills and shortages of others, or it may facilitate the absorption of new workers (through better labour market communication systems, for example), the conversion of old capital stock, and so on. Moreover, one can ask the question (unfortunately without being able to answer it with much confidence) of whether population change tends to increase or decrease the rate of technological advance.

The types of adjustment just discussed are closely related to the issue of changes in industrial structure. Indeed, changes in the patterns of demand for goods imply pressures on some industries to expand and others to contract. How fast can the industrial structure adjust to these pressures? Demographic changes may imply changes in the geographic distribution of the population, and one can also ask how fast the geographic distribution of industry can respond – or, since the relationships run in both directions, how fast the distribution of population can respond to the redistribution of industry. Population change and economic responses to it clearly have an important geographic dimension.

Last, but by no means least in importance in the list of adjustment problems or processes, are the social and political ones. Of particular relevance for the present purpose are the questions of how fast, and to what extent, society and its elected governments will respond to the altered patterns of demand for public services implied by population aging. How fast will public opinion or government initiative respond to the requirements for budgetary reallocations (among education, health care, and pensions, especially) and the associated requirements for tax revenues and changes in intergovernmental revenue-sharing arrangements?

THE ARITHMETIC OF INTERGENERATIONAL DEPENDENCY

Some of the basic economic implications of changes in population structure can be inferred simply from the population itself, or from the population and the labour force. Various dependency ratios can be calculated and the changes in them through time observed. Some such ratios are displayed in Table 3. Other ratios can be defined, but in fact it makes no difference for our

TABLE 3: Alternative Measures of Dependency in the Canadian Population: Historical 1921–81; Projected 1991–2051

	Dependency ratios based on population age structure				Dependency ratios based on labour force and population	
Year	Pop. 0–19 / Pop. 20–64	Pop. 65+ / Pop. 20–64	Pop. 0–19 and 65+ / Pop. 20–64	Total pop. / Pop. 20–64	Non-labour force / Labour force	Total pop. / Labour force
1921	.84	.09	.94	1.94	1.68	2.68
1931	.79	.10	.89	1.89	1.59	2.59
1941	.67	.12	.79	1.79	1.50	2.50
1951	.70	.14	.84	1.84	1.62	2.62
1961	.83	.15	.98	1.98	1.75	2.75
1971	.75	.15	.90	1.90	1.47	2.47
1981	.55	.17	.72	1.72	1.00	2.00
			Standard			
1991	.46	.19	.64	1.64	.89	1.89
2001	.42	.20	.62	1.62	.82	1.82
2011	.37	.22	.59	1.59	.83	1.83
2021	.37	.29	.66	1.66	.94	1.94
2031	.38	.38	.76	1.76	1.02	2.02
2041	.37	.39	.76	1.76	1.02	2.02
2051	.37	.39	.76	1.76	1.03	2.03
			High Fertility			
1991	.54	.19	.73	1.73	.99	1.99
2001	.65	.20	.85	1.85	1.06	2.06
2011	.62	.20	.82	1.82	1.03	2.03
2021	.66	.24	.90	1.90	1.13	2.13
2031	.72	.28	1.00	2.00	1.17	2.17
2041	.69	.23	.92	1.92	1.09	2.09
2051	.69	.20	.90	1.90	1.10	2.10

			Low Fertility			
1991	.44	.19	.63	1.63	.87	1.87
2001	.38	.20	.58	1.58	.78	1.78
2011	.32	.22	.55	1.55	.80	1.80
2021	.32	.30	.62	1.62	.91	1.91
2031	.32	.41	.73	1.73	1.01	2.01
2041	.32	.43	.75	1.75	1.04	2.04
2051	.32	.45	.77	1.77	1.05	2.05

purposes. All of the alternative ratios that one might calculate tell the same basic story about the past and the likely future.

Let us take the populations under the age of twenty and sixty-five years of age and over as "dependent," and the population in between as "economically active." This is a crude approximation, of course, but it serves our purposes well enough. On this basis, the first two columns of Table 3 show child and elderly dependency ratios, respectively, and the third shows the overall dependency ratio, defined as the ratio of the combined populations under twenty and sixty-five and over to the population twenty to sixty-four. Alternatively, we may define the overall dependency ratio as the ratio of the *total* population to the population twenty to sixty-four – the total number of mouths to be fed as a ratio to the number of "providers," so to speak.

The child dependency ratio reached its post-World War II peak at the beginning of the 1960s, although even then it was no higher than it had been in the early 1920s. Since 1961 or thereabouts it has declined very sharply: from 0.83 persons under twenty for every person twenty to sixty-four in 1961, the ratio had fallen to 0.55 by 1981. Barring a resumption of higher fertility levels, it can be expected to fall to 0.46 or lower by 1991, and perhaps to about 0.37 by the year 2011 (based on the standard projection). One might expect, therefore, a continuing decline in the fraction of the national product required for education and the support of the young population generally. (We are referring to demographic effects, of course; non-demographic influences are another matter.)

Declines in the child dependency ratio will be offset by increases in the elderly dependency ratio. The latter increases will be relatively small and gradual for the next three decades or so, but then quite rapid in the second and third decades of the next century as the children of the baby boom complete their working lives and move into the retirement ages. From 0.17 in 1981, the elderly ratio rises to 0.39 by 2041, according to the standard projection. Unquestionably this implies a very large increase in the resources to be devoted to the support of the elderly.

Combining the two ratios into a single dependency ratio suggests that the overall "dependency burden" will not increase in the next several decades; even by 2051, the overall ratio will be well below levels of 1961 and 1971. As always, this assumes no return to high fertility. However, even in the high projection, the maximum overall dependency ratios are virtually the same as those of 1961, and they are not reached for some five decades.

The same picture emerges if we redefine the overall dependency ratios in terms of population and labour force. The last two columns of Table 3 show ratios of non-labour force to labour force and total population to labour force, respectively. As before, the projected ratios never come near the levels of the 1950s, the 1960s, and early 1970s. In fact, even in the high fertility projection, the labour force-based ratios fall well short of these historical levels. Whatever implications the future aging of the population may have for the Canadian economy, the overall dependency burden is not likely to be excessive, by historical standards. The problems will be those of shifting resources from old uses to new ones as the population age structure evolves, rather than any overall "lack" of resources.

A SIMPLE MODEL AND SOME SIMULATIONS OF THE EFFECTS OF POPULATION CHANGE ON THE NATIONAL PRODUCT

While it is clear that population and labour force change of the magnitude just discussed will have a substantial impact on the macroeconomy, the potential magnitude of that impact cannot be foretold a priori. Instead, a framework or model is needed, in which to take account of both demand and supply effects. A schematic representation of such a model is provided in Figure 1. (Not all of the effects discussed above are reflected in this model; in the interest of simplicity, only the more important ones are provided for.)

Changes in the overall size and age-sex distribution of the population occur in response to births, deaths, immigration, and emigration, as indicated in the left side of the figure. The labour force, in turn, is drawn from the population. Migration has an immediate impact on labour force size and age

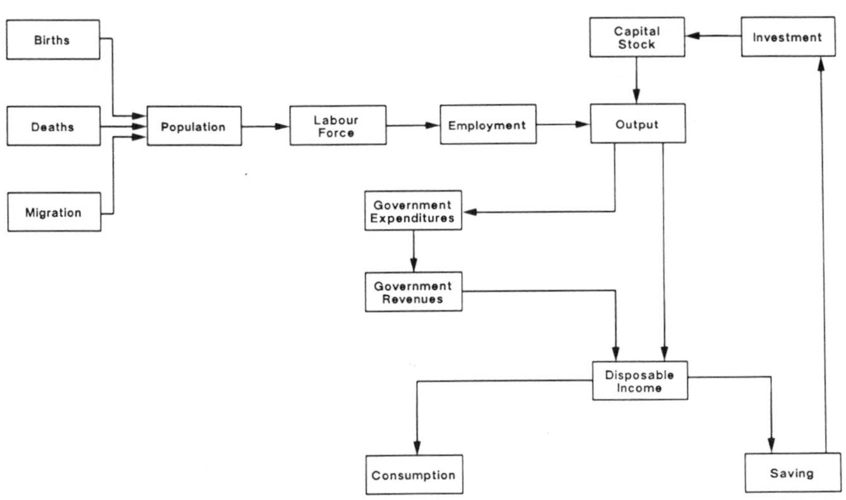

FIGURE 1: Schematic representation of the economic-demographic system

composition, since many migrants are of labour force age at the time of their move, whereas newborn children reach labour force age only with a lag of one and a half to two decades. Deaths occur at all ages, of course, but in most developed economies relatively few occur among those of labour force age.

Employment is determined by the size of the labour force, after allowance for unemployment, and, together with the available capital stock, determines the productive capacity of the economy. Each year the government draws off some of the output and uses it to purchase commodities and services and to effect transfer payments within the population. In the model of Figure 1, such purchases and transfers are paid for out of tax revenues and the government budget is always in balance. What remains is the aggregate disposable income of the community. It is allocated between current consumption expenditure on the one hand and saving on the other. The savings are used, through the vehicle of investment expenditures, to add to the nation's capital stock, and hence to its productive capacity in subsequent periods.

The model depicted in broad outline in Figure 1 has been specified mathematically and embodied in a computer programme designed for projections or simulation analysis. The programme keeps track of the population, labour force, and employment by single years of age, separately for men and women, and it moves the entire economic-demographic system ahead year by year in simulated time for as many years as desired. Even though it embodies considerable detail, the model is clearly highly stylized. It abstracts from a number of issues of importance in the shorter term (such as inflation and unemployment) in order to focus attention on some of the more fundamental longer-term consequences of demographic change.[3]

Some illustrative projections (or "simulated futures") based on this model are provided in Table 4. The projections start with a population and labour force having the age and sex characteristics of the 1981 Canadian population. The projections are based on the standard demographic and labour force assumptions described in the section on the Canadian population and labour force.

The second two columns in the upper part of Table 4 show the projected population and labour force for the period 1981 to 2051. (The numbers here are in index form, with 1981 equal to 100.0, but are otherwise identical to those in the standard projections reported in Table 1.) The next three columns show indexes of "potential output" – that is, the output which the economic system as a whole is capable of producing with sustained high employment of human and capital resources. Clearly the growth of potential output depends on the assumed rate of technical progress or productivity increase, and we explore three alternative growth scenarios – slow, medium, and high. "Slow" is defined by a zero rate of technical progress, "medium" by a rate of one per cent per year, and "high" by a rate of two per cent per year.

TABLE 4: Population, Labour Force, and Potential Output under Alternative Assumptions about the Rate of Productivity Growth, 1981–2051, Based on Standard Population and Labour Force Projections

			Potential output		
Year	Population	Labour force	Slow growth	Medium growth	High growth
			Index: 1981–100		
1981	100.0	100.0	100.0	100.0	100.0
1991	111.1	117.7	113.1	120.7	128.5
2001	119.6	131.4	123.8	141.2	160.6
2011	125.8	137.3	130.1	159.8	196.2
2021	130.2	134.5	130.4	174.2	232.8
2031	131.6	130.5	128.1	187.5	274.6
2041	130.2	128.7	127.0	203.9	327.5
2051	127.3	125.5	124.9	220.5	389.5
			% rates of growth		
1991	1.1	1.6	1.2	1.9	2.5
2001	.7	1.1	.9	1.6	2.3
2011	.5	.4	.5	1.2	2.0
2021	.3	–.2	.0	.9	1.7
2031	.1	–.3	–.2	.7	1.7
2041	–.1	–.1	–.1	.8	1.8
2051	–.2	–.3	–.2	.8	1.7
			Per capita		
1981	—	—	100.0	100.0	100.0
1991	—	—	101.8	108.6	115.6
2001	—	—	103.5	118.0	134.2
2011	—	—	103.4	127.1	156.0
2021	—	—	100.1	133.8	178.8
2031	—	—	97.4	142.5	208.7
2041	—	—	97.6	156.6	251.6
2051	—	—	98.1	173.2	305.9

Note: Growth rates refer to the decade preceding each of the indicated years.

(It may be noted that the estimated rate in Canada over the decade ending in 1983 was close to zero, while over the period 1927–83 it was about 2.2 per cent. See Denton and Spencer 1985.) The middle and lower parts of the table repeat the upper portion, but in terms of annual average rates of growth of potential output and levels of potential output per capita.

Consider first the slow growth scenario. In this case, output increases are due entirely to increases in the labour force. However, whereas the labour force grows from its base value of 100.0 in 1981 to a peak of 137.3 in 2011, output grows to only 130.1 in that year, and attains its own somewhat higher peak a decade later. In this projection, the labour force grows faster than potential output in the first two decades and somewhat more slowly thereafter, a result that is largely attributable to changes in the age distribution of the labour force. In 1981 the labour force had been growing very rapidly for two decades, and hence was very young on average. Even though labour force growth will be much less rapid during the remainder of the 1980s and throughout the 1990s, it will nonetheless continue to be substantial and to outstrip general economic growth. In our model, however, as the labour force ages it can also be expected to become more productive, as its members gain experience. Thus the future absolute drop in the level of potential output commences later than the labour force reduction in the slow growth scenario, and is more gradual.

If there is any significant degree of effective technical progress, potential output can be expected to grow more rapidly than the labour force and to yield increasing levels of output per capita. This is evident from the last two columns. In the medium growth scenario, output per capita would increase by 18 per cent by the end of this century, compared to only 3.5 per cent in the slow growth scenario and 34.2 per cent in the high growth scenario; by the middle of the next century it would have increased by 73 per cent with medium growth, compared to a decrease of almost 2 per cent under the slow growth assumption and an increase of more than 200 per cent under the high growth assumption. This very wide range of possibilities shows clearly the importance of the rate of technical progress in productivity growth for future per capita income levels.

EFFECTS ON GOVERNMENT EXPENDITURES

As individuals age, their claims on and contributions to the public treasury change considerably. People go to publicly funded schools while young, receive support under national pension plans while old, and benefit from publicly funded health care services at all ages, but especially at older ages, when health care costs are much higher on average. Thus we might expect that major changes in the population age distribution would result in correspondingly large changes in the claims made upon such publicly funded services, and that this would be reflected in greater government revenue requirements and higher rates of taxation.

Working at a highly disaggregated level, we have attempted to estimate the impact which future population changes might be expected to have on public expenditures, on the assumption that the quality of public services remains constant over the next several decades. By "constant quality" we mean that the level of expenditure per capita for each age-sex group remains unchanged over time in real (price-adjusted) terms. (The results are reported

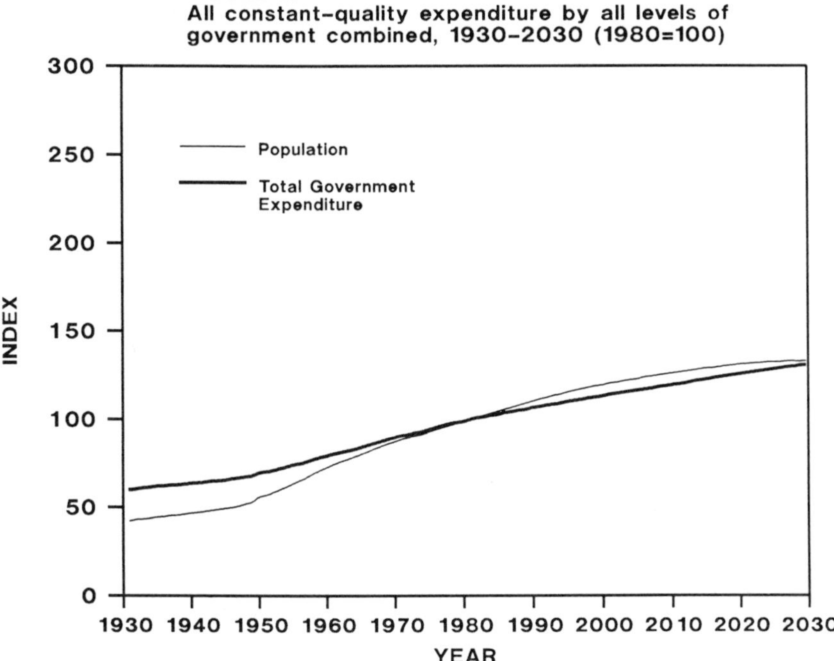

in more detail in Denton and Spencer 1985; here they are merely summarized briefly.)

Figure 2 shows indexes of population and constant-quality government expenditure in total for the period 1930–2030. We observe that over the period from 1930 to 1980 the population (indicated by the dotted line) increased more than did total constant-quality government expenditures (indicated by the solid line); the same observation holds true for most of the projection period from 1980 to 2030, although by 2030 the accumulated proportionate increases over 1980 levels are about the same for the two series.

The picture is quite different for particular components of expenditure. We single out for illustration the three expenditure categories that are most sensitive to demographic change – namely social security, health care, and education.

The greatest of the population-induced increases by far is in the category of social security (which includes the Canada Pension Plan, the Quebec Pension Plan, and Old Age Security). The implications of maintaining a constant-quality expenditure level for these programs is illustrated in Figure 3. The inevitable rise in the number of older people causes an increase of almost 30 per cent in social security costs between 1980 and 1990, and of more

FIGURE 3:
Constant-quality expenditure on social security by all levels of government combined, 1930-2030 (1980=100)

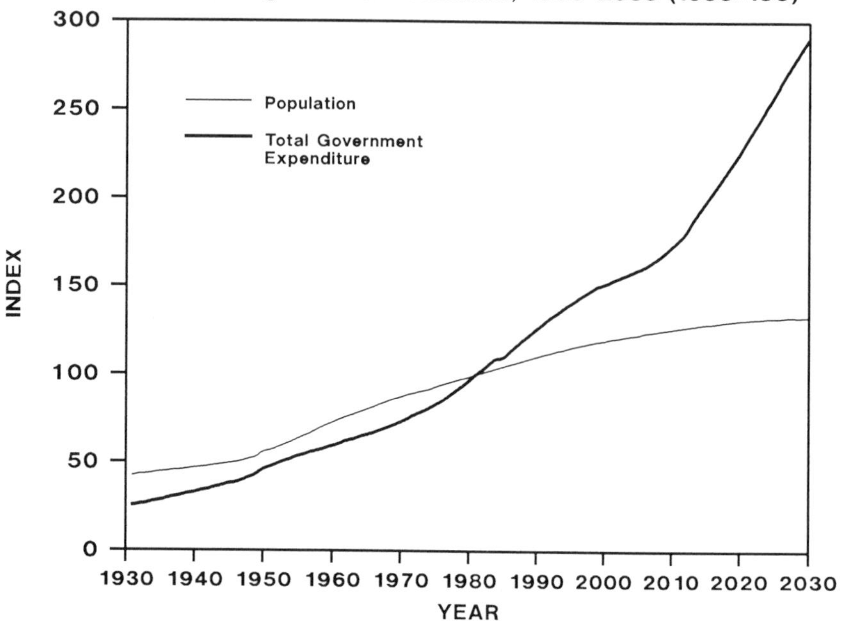

FIGURE 4:
Constant-quality expenditure on health care by all levels of government combined, 1930-2030 (1980=100)

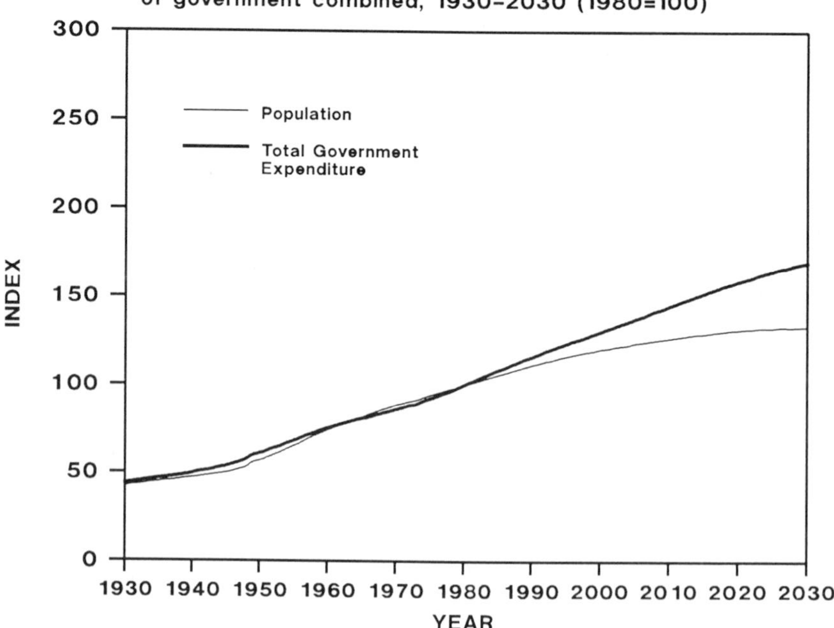

than 50 per cent by 2000. By the year 2030, social security costs are roughly three times their 1980 levels. Under present institutional arrangements, the costs of social security in Canada are going to rise very sharply in this decade and in the ones to follow.

The category that shows the second-greatest rates of increase is health, illustrated in Figure 4. Under the standard projection, health expenditures increase by 16.2 per cent over the whole of the fifty-year period. The reason for the marked increase in health costs is, of course, the tendency for rates of utilization to rise sharply with age. Increasing health costs, like increasing social security costs, will be one of the manifestations of the process of population aging in Canada.

Again under the assumptions of the standard projection, education costs will fall in this decade and will be lower throughout the fifty-year projection period than they were in 1980. This is true both of elementary and secondary education and of post-secondary and other education, as illustrated in Figures 5 and 6.

Thus we can anticipate that the big increases in government expenditures resulting from future demographic changes will be in social security and health and the decreases will be in education. In most of the other categories of expenditure, there will be some increases but these will be modest and below the rate of growth of the population.

INCOME SUPPORT FOR THE ELDERLY

The simultaneous effects of demographic change on both the productive capacity of the economy and the claims for particular categories of expenditure can be analysed with the use of an economic-demographic macro-model of the kind discussed earlier. The model can be modified to incorporate a "pension sector," a "health care sector," and an "education sector" to keep track of the expenditure implications for costs of each kind, and the costs can be compared with the economy's overall productive capacity – that is, with the ability to "meet the costs."

Our intention here is not to model closely actual conditions in the Canadian economy, but rather to illustrate the general nature of the impacts associated with population change alone. In the case of pension costs, we characterize the overall social security system with the assumption that each person of age sixty-five or over receives a transfer payment equal in value to one-quarter of the average wage. This is at best a very rough approximation of the actual situation, which includes among the public-source income support for the elderly the Canada Pension Plan (under the provisions of which individuals may receive at most a pension payment equal to one-quarter the average industrial wage), Old Age Assistance, and the Old Age Supplement. However, the approximation suffices for our present illustrative purpose.

FIGURE 5:
Constant-quality expenditure on elementary and secondary education by all levels of government combined, 1930-2030 (1980=100)

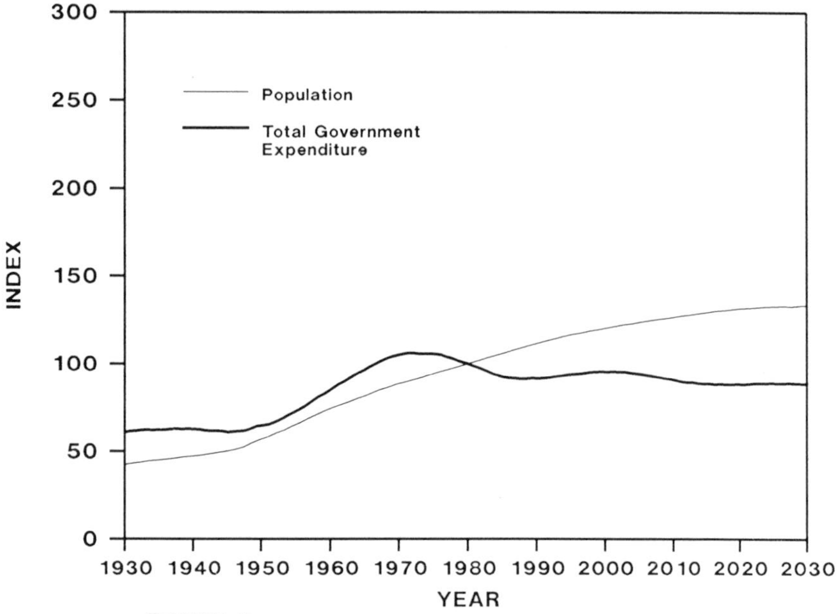

FIGURE 6:
Constant-quality expenditure on postsecondary and "other" education by all levels of government combined, 1930-2030 (1980=100)

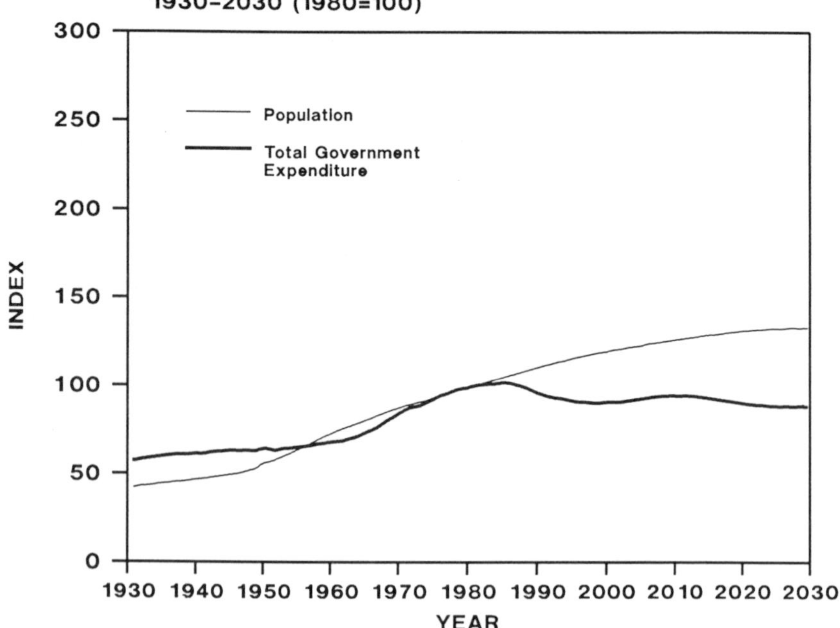

TABLE 5: Projected Pension, Health-Care, and Education Costs Relative to the Productive Capacity of the Economy, 1981–2051, Based on Standard Population Projection

Year	Pension costs	Health-care costs	Education costs	Total
		% of potential output		
1981	3.4	7.0	7.5	17.9
1991	3.7	7.2	6.0	16.9
2001	3.9	7.4	5.6	16.9
2011	4.4	7.8	5.1	17.4
2021	5.9	8.5	4.9	19.4
2031	7.6	9.2	5.0	21.9
2041	7.8	9.5	4.9	22.1
2051	7.7	9.4	4.8	22.0

As can be seen from the second column of Table 5, the age-sex structure of the population in 1981 implied a commitment of 3.4 per cent of the productive capacity of the economy in that year, under the assumptions that we have made. Taken in conjunction with the standard population and labour force projections, this proportion would rise to 3.9 per cent by the turn of the century, to 5.9 per cent by 2021 (when those born early in the baby boom will have reached age sixty-five), and to 7.8 per cent by 2041 (by which year all members of the baby boom generation will be in old age).

An important question is what would happen if population growth were either more rapid or less rapid than under our standard assumptions. It turns out that future population growth and pension costs are much more sensitive to assumptions about the birth rate than to assumptions about mortality or migration rates. (See, for example, Denton and Spencer 1981). With this in mind, we report projections based on the high and low fertility assumptions discussed in the section on Canadian population and labour force. The results for pension costs are reported in the first column of Tables 6 and 7. Pension costs are seen to rise by the same amount by the turn of the century, whatever the fertility assumption. Thereafter the costs continue to rise under both the high and low assumptions. However, we see that by 2031 only 5.2 per cent of productive capacity is required to meet pension commitments under the high assumption compared to 8.3 per cent under the low one. The difference is explained largely by the relationship between the population in old age and that in labour force age: with high fertility there would be only 28 people over age sixty-five for every 100 people aged twenty to sixty-four, compared to 41 per 100 under the assumption of low fertility. However, in all cases it is clear that over the next half-century we should expect a substantial increase in the costs of maintaining our current pension system.

HEALTH CARE COSTS

Similar projections have been made for the health care sector, and are reported in the third columns of Tables 5 through 7. Once again, the assumption underlying these projections is that the quality of health care services will be maintained, in the sense that individuals at each age will continue to receive, on average, the same allocation of real health care resources as in 1981.[4]

In 1981 health care costs accounted for approximately 7 per cent of the gross national product, and this has been taken as the starting value. Under the standard projection, the proportion rises slightly by the turn of the century (to 7.4 per cent) and more sharply thereafter, reaching 9.2 in 2031 and a peak of 9.5 per cent in 2041. Alternative fertility assumptions are of some importance: health care costs would rise more rapidly over the next few decades with a return to relatively high fertility levels than with a continuation of low levels. The reason is the high costs of health care associated with pregnancy, birth, and the first year of life. For example, by 2001 projected health care costs are 7.2 per cent under the low fertility assumption, compared to 8.2 per cent under the high assumption. However, the difference eventually diminishes, and then disappears altogether by 2051.

EDUCATION COSTS

It is estimated that in 1981 approximately 7.5 per cent of the gross national product was allocated to education, and we take that as our starting value. We then assess the overall cost implications of maintaining the 1981 levels of real educational resources allocated to individuals of various ages, under the alternative population assumptions. An element of the constant-quality assumption is that the age-specific educational enrolment rates remain at their 1981 levels: any change in these rates would represent a change in quality, as defined here.

The cost implications are reported in the fourth columns of Tables 5 through 7. Education costs associated with population change can be expected to decline, relative to productive capacity, unless there is a return to high fertility levels. For example, education costs would fall by 1.9 percentage points (to 5.6 per cent of capacity) by 2001 under the standard fertility assumption, and by somewhat more under the low assumption, whereas under the high assumption such costs would rise slightly. Over the longer term the differences are much more substantial: five decades from now, constant-quality education costs would represent less than half the claim on productive capacity with low fertility than they would with high fertility.

TABLE 6: Projected Pension, Health-Care, and Education Costs Relative to the Productive Capacity of the Economy, 1981–2051, Based on High Fertility Population Projection

Year	Pension costs	Health-care costs	Education costs	Total
		% of potential output		
1981	3.4	7.0	7.5	17.9
1991	3.7	7.2	6.3	17.8
2001	3.9	8.2	7.6	19.6
2011	3.9	8.7	8.1	20.8
2021	4.7	9.4	8.2	22.4
2031	5.2	9.7	9.3	24.2
2041	4.4	9.7	9.2	23.3
2051	3.9	9.6	9.3	22.8

TABLE 7: Projected Pension, Health-Care, and Education Costs Relative to the Productive Capacity of the Economy, 1981–2051, Based on Low Fertility Population Projection

Year	Pension costs	Health-care costs	Education costs	Total
		% of potential output		
1981	3.4	7.0	7.5	17.9
1991	3.7	7.1	6.0	16.8
2001	3.9	7.2	5.3	16.5
2011	4.5	7.7	4.6	16.7
2021	6.2	8.5	4.3	19.0
2031	8.3	9.2	4.3	21.8
2041	8.8	9.6	4.1	22.5
2051	9.0	9.6	4.1	22.7

CONCLUSION

The age structure of the Canadian population is changing markedly and will continue to change in the decades ahead. Undoubtedly this will result in social and political tensions and will raise important ethical issues relating to the allocation of the nation's resources – to "who gets what." However, the economic effects of population aging are often not well understood. There will be pressure on government budgets in some areas, but the economy's productive capacity, and hence its tax base, will also increase. Even simple calculations of population dependency ratios suggest that the "burden" of increased proportions of elderly dependents will be offset in large measure by the smaller proportions of child dependents and higher proportions of the population in the working ages. In all likelihood, the future ratios of dependent to working population will be well below the levels of the 1950s, 1960s, and early 1970s; only a very large increase in the birth rate would produce dependency ratios comparable to those earlier ones.

The slowing down of population growth implies, of course,a slower rate of economic expansion, other things being equal. However, the growth of productivity is a critical factor, and one that may be far more important than any demographic considerations in determining future levels of potential output and income.

Demographic forces will certainly tend to drive up pension and health care costs, but at the same time they will tend to drive down the costs of education – unless, of course, there is a return to higher levels of fertility. Overall, it seems likely that government expenditures as a share of the potential gross national product will rise little or not at all as a consequence of population change until well into the next century, and when there are increases they will be of relatively small proportion. The important economic problems associated with the population aging in the decades ahead will have to do much more with the *reallocation* of resources than with any insufficiency of overall resources to meet changing demands. That is not to suggest that problems of adjustment or reallocation are easy problems to deal with, but it is perhaps comforting to know that (at least in economic terms) they should be manageable ones.

NOTES

1 This paper was prepared for presentation at the Symposium on Ethics and Aging, University of British Columbia, 16–19 August 1984. The assistance of Christine Feaver in the programming of the model and computer simulations reported here is acknowledge gratefully. Financial support from the Social Sciences and Humanities Research Council of Canada under the terms of a strategic grant awarded jointly to the authors and to Victor W. Marshall has made possible our continuing research program on the economic and social implications of an aging population.

2 A detailed description of the approach used, along with a number of detailed projections, is available in Denton, Feaver, and Spencer (1980).

3 The interested reader will find a detailed description of similar economic-demographic models in Denton and Spencer (1973, 1975a).

4 Health care costs are high at birth and during the first few months of life; thereafter they decline until about age ten, after which they rise with age, at first gradually and then more steeply, reaching very high average levels in old age. A detailed account of the age-cost profile and a fuller analysis of the cost implications associated with population change are provided in Denton and Spencer (1975b, 1983a, 1983b).

REFERENCES

Denton, F.T., Feaver, C.H., & Spencer, B.G. (1980). *The future population and labour force of Canada: Projections to the year 2051*. Ottawa: Economic Council of Canada

Denton, F.T., & Spencer, B.G. (1973). A simulation analysis of the effects of population change on a neoclassical economy. *Journal of Political Economy, 81*, 356–75

———. (1975a). *Population and the economy*. Lexington, MA: D.C. Heath

———. (1975b). Health-care costs when the population changes. *Canadian Journal of Economics, 8*, 34–48

———. (1981). A macroeconomic analysis of the effects of a public pension plan. *Canadian Journal of Economics, 14*, 609–34

———. (1983a). Population aging and future health costs in Canada. *Canadian Public Policy, 9*, 155–63

———. (1983b). The sensitivity of health-care costs to changes in population age structure. In Christopher Garbacz (Ed.), *Economic resources for the elderly: Prospects for the future*. Boulder, CO: Westview Press

———. (1985). Prospective changes in the population and their implications for government expenditures. In T.J. Courchene, D.W. Conklin, and G.C.A. Cook (Eds.), *Ottawa and the provinces: The distribution of money and power*. Toronto: Ontario Economic Council

PART TWO

Specific Issues

9

The Right to Participate: Ending Discrimination Against the Elderly

DONALD J. MACDOUGALL

It is not unusual for people working in the health professions or social services to view elderly people as consumers of these services. Asked to consider ethical issues affecting the elderly, they are likely to respond in terms of their own special expertise. Serious ethical questions do arise in those areas and several papers in this volume deal with those questions.

There is, however, a danger in the "medicalization" of the debate. There are broader ethical issues that should be discussed. For example, what restrictions, if any, can be justifiably imposed on the individual in order to advance the common good? In particular, can compulsory retirement at a specified age be justified? What obligations do the younger generations have to the elderly? What obligations do the elderly have to the younger generations? Is planning for old age a matter of individual, family, and/or state responsibility – and how is the responsibility of each determined?

We shy away from these broader ethical issues. There is a natural bias in favour of the status quo. Communities tend to accept existing social and cultural practices as inherently right. Politicians, scholars, and bureaucrats, who may know better, may be sceptical about their ability to influence social change until the public perceives that a crisis is developing and that action is necessary. The dramatic demographic changes predicted in the near future seem certain to challenge that complacency and provoke a debate about the broader ethical issues.

At the heart of the debate will be the relationship between the individual and society, especially the relationship between the individual and the state – an issue that continues to engage the intellects of both legal and political philosophers. At one extreme you have anarchism – the maximization of individual autonomy. At the other extreme you have the welfare state – whether Marxist or capitalist – with its emphasis on social goals rather than individual freedom.

Bentham's utilitarian ethics provided a theoretical foundation for the modern welfare state as it has developed in the British Commonwealth and the United States. He contemplated an active legislature. And every measure of government, as well as every action of a private individual, was to be judged by whether it augmented or diminished the happiness of the society in question: "Now private ethics has happiness for its end: and legislation can have no other. Private ethics concerns every member; that is, the happiness and the actions of every member, of any community that can be proposed; and legislation can concern no more. Thus far, then, private ethics and the art of legislation go hand in hand."[1] However, he did qualify this general position. He suggested that the coercive powers of the law should not be exercised where punishment would be groundless, inefficacious, unprofitable, or needless.

But these qualifications were not sufficient to silence modern critics. Recently H. L. A. Hart (1976) commented:

> Utilitarianism, which for long was regarded as the sober workmanlike English manifestation of the European Enlightenment and which was certainly the fountain of great reforms of the archaic English system as well as the inspiration of progressive thought in England and elsewhere, is now seen by many thinkers to have a darker, more sinister side, licensing anything to be done to individuals, condoning any sacrifice, in the pursuit of the ultimate goal of maximizing the aggregate or average welfare of a community.[2]

Some modern American political philosophers – such as John Rawls[3] and Robert Nozick[4] – emphasize that society is composed of a large number of separate individuals and suggest that an individual may have an ethical right to pursue certain interests even if maintaining his right to do so may reduce the level of aggregate or average welfare below that which could otherwise be achieved. Rawls, for example, sets out as his first principle of justice: "Each person is to have an equal right to the most extensive total system of equal basic liberties compatible with a similar system of liberty for all."[5]

This controversy about the appropriate balance between individual liberty and the common good is central to all the ethical issues raised by our treatment of the elderly. To make the broader ethical issues more concrete, I want to illustrate them by discussing three specific issues – age discrimination, compulsory retirement, and income security for older Canadians.

AGE DISCRIMINATION

Approximately 10 per cent of the population is aged sixty-five or over. That percentage will increase significantly after 1990 and even more sharply after 2010, as the baby boom generation reaches sixty-five. Canada's aging population will put pressure on her health care and social service delivery systems, and it is natural for people to be concerned with those issues. But many of the elderly will be basically healthy, and even those who are not may wish to pursue activities within the limitations imposed by their health. Yet most of Canada's older people will suffer discrimination because of their age. In some cases this will be a reflection of social attitudes. In other cases (for example, compulsory retirement), social practices have been incorporated into legal rules.

What is the interest that is infringed upon by these social and legal practices? In a brief to the Manitoba Commission on Compulsory Retirement (1982), the Manitoba Human Rights Commission phrased the issue in these terms:

> From a human rights perspective there is perhaps no better example of the arbitrary treatment of individuals in the defined group than is the case with mandatory retirement. The whole essence of human rights philosophy is that a person be treated as an individual and not considered necessarily to exhibit the same behaviour or attitude as other members within his or her identifiable group. . . in short the emphasis should be on accepting the reality of individual differences *and the freedom of the individual to make a choice*.[6]

Similarly, the *Report of the Parliamentary Committee on Equality Rights* (1985) stated:

> Mandatory retirement is a classic example of the denial of equality on improper grounds. It involves the arbitrary treatment of individuals simply because they are members of an identifiable group. Mandatory retirement does not allow for consideration of individual characteristics, even though those caught by the rule are likely to display a wide variety of the capabilities relevant to employment. It is an easy way of being selective that is based, in whole or in part, on stereotypical assumptions about the performance of older workers.[7]

It is not surprising that the law has been invoked to combat age discrimination. In the United States there are two key acts: the Age Discrimination in

Employment Act and the Age Discrimination Act. The Age Discrimination in Employment Act prevents employers from using age as the basis for employment decisions – effectively eliminating compulsory retirement. The Age Discrimination Act bars discrimination on the basis of age in any federally supported program, unless that program was specifically designated for a particular age group.

In Canada the Charter of Rights and Freedoms contains a provision that prohibits age discrimination (section 15). That provision came into force in April 1985 and states: "Every individual is equal before and under the law and has the right to equal protection and equal benefit of the law without discrimination and, in particular, without discrimination based on race, national or ethnic origin, religion, sex, *age* or mental or physical disability."[8]

It is difficult to assess what impact this provision will have. First, the Charter applies only to governments (section 32). Thus section 15 will not affect private, non-governmental discrimination. Second, section 15 is "subject only to such reasonable limits prescribed by law as can be demonstrably justified in a free and democratic society" (section 1). Third, the provinces have the power to override this provision of the Charter (section 33). Lastly, section 15 does not invalidate legislation that has as its objective the amelioration of conditions for persons in the protected group.

It would be foolhardy for anyone at this stage to predict how effective section 15 of the Charter will be in protecting the liberty of the elderly. The early cases have been concerned with the distinction between governmental and non-governmental actions. In *Stoffman* v. *Vancouver General Hospital*[9] the British Columbia Supreme Court decided that the hospital was an agency of the provincial government because the government effectively controlled its affairs. Thus hospital regulations which terminated, at age sixty-five, the plaintiff doctor's admitting privileges offended section 15 of the Charter. However, universities and school boards have been regarded as independent of government, so that the Charter has no significance for their mandatory retirement policies.[10] In at least one case, *Re McKinney and the University of Guelph,*[11] the Court took the view that even if the university's mandatory retirement policy was discriminatory under section 15 of the Charter, it could be justified under section 1. Section 1 provides criteria justifying certain limits on the rights and freedoms guaranteed by the Charter. The Court was satisfied (1) that the university's mandatory retirement policy had important objectives; (2) that the method of implementation was rationally connected to those objectives; and (3) that the policy did not have a disproportionate effect on the rights protected by section 15 of the Charter.

Most of these decisions are under appeal and it may be some time before the effect of section 15 can be determined. But the indications are that section

15 will have a limited impact on the way the elderly are treated in our society. In many situations it will be inapplicable because there is no government action involved. Even where section 15 applies, the government may find it relatively easy to justify discrimination under section 1 of the Charter. Indeed Justice Gray stated in *Re McKinney and the University of Guelph:* "There is much to be said for the respondent's submission that the nature of the right at issue here – freedom from discrimination based on age – is less sensitive than the other rights enumerated in section 15(1) of the Charter."[12] The other significant Canadian legal protection against discrimination is contained in the provincial Human Rights acts or codes. To evaluate their effectiveness, it is useful to examine how effectively they protect the individual's right to continue working when he has the capacity and desire to do so.

COMPULSORY RETIREMENT

There has been considerable research into the factors that influence *voluntary* retirement. Clearly the individual's health, working conditions, and financial resources are key considerations. But what is the basis of the compulsory retirement policies that affect more than 75 per cent of employees of large organizations?[13]

William Graebner, in his book *A History of Retirement,*[14] suggested that the initial push, in the late nineteenth century, came from industrialists concerned with productivity and efficiency. Although later studies demonstrated that older workers were often more productive than younger ones,[15] employers continued to favour younger workers – and, as the economy entered the depression of the 1930s, retirement seemed an appropriate remedy for unemployment in depressed industries. Moreover, compulsory retirement permitted an employer to replace expensive senior workers with inexpensive junior workers. And automatic retirement schemes provided an alternative to the development of detailed performance standards. Indeed, many critics of compulsory retirement consider that management's desire to avoid hard decisions was the main reason why compulsory retirement became the norm. Charles E. Odell (1977) testified before the U.S. Senate Committee on Human Resources that "we simply lack the will to bring about the basic changes. We go on encouraging the lazy man's way of handling the problem – drop everyone at a fixed age and avoid having to explain why some, if they choose, can go on working."[16]

Four factors mentioned by Graebner still operate to sustain compulsory retirement schemes. They are: (1) concern for efficiency and productivity, (2) concern about the unemployment of the younger worker, (3) employment costs, and (4) avoidance of evaluation.

However, it would have been difficult to "sell" retirement without accompanying pension schemes. Graebner took the position that retirement was sold. He commented:

> Between 1940 and 1965, retirement triumphed over alternative methods of dealing with the aged. This was in part a mechanical process. Pension plans grew in numbers and coverage, social security was extended to additional elements of the work force, while benefits were increased and retirement ages lowered. As this process met with resistance, the leading advocates and beneficiaries of retirement – corporations, labour unions, and insurance companies – became increasingly aggressive in marketing retirement as a consumable commodity, ignoring its origins as a device for corporate and bureaucratic efficiency and control. . . . They were assisted by a group of sociologists whose concept of "disengagement" affirmed the existence of a natural process by which the aged separated themselves from the workplace and other primary institutions.[17]

Other commentators have given a less conspiratorial explanation of developments in that period. W. Andrew Achenbaum (1983) emphasized the rising emphasis on leisure activities and retirement as a "well deserved and earned release from the instrumental chores of work."[18] These were the forces that ensured that compulsory retirement became the norm in North America – despite its unfairness to some individuals and its social disadvantages.

In the United States, the Age Discrimination in Employment Act, first passed in 1967 but amended several times since, prohibits employers from using age as a basis for employment decisions. A 1978 amendment protected employees under the age of seventy. A 1986 amendment removed that "cap" so that the act now protects employees over seventy. There are some exceptions. Thus the legislation exempts police officers, firefighters, tenured university faculty, and executives with annual pensions of $44,000 or more.

In Canada, provincial human rights legislation generally prohibits age discrimination in employment – but often defines age to "mean an age of 45 years or more and less than 65 years." Consequently such legislation gives no protection to a person over sixty-five. The clear exceptions to this are Manitoba and Quebec. The Manitoba Human Rights Act contains an open-ended prohibition against discrimination because of age in employment (section 6) and it has been invoked by several people who were retired, against their wishes, at sixty-five: a university professor,[19] a civil servant,[20] a neurosurgeon,[21] an assembler,[22] and a schoolteacher.[23]

The case of the neurosurgeon is particularly interesting. Consider the position of the hospital. If it terminated his right to use the hospital facilities, it faced a suit brought by the neurosurgeon. But if he was permitted to continue in practice and any of his treatment was challenged, a lawyer would certainly argue that the hospital was negligent in permitting him to continue as a neurosurgeon. The critical issue, in law and in ethics, is the capacity of the individual. But there may be little direct evidence available concerning that – so the issue is likely to be blurred by discussions of averages and probabilities.

A major defence to a charge of age discrimination in employment is that the age qualification is a "bona fide occupational requirement" or "reasonable occupational qualification."[24] In essence, the defence is that for certain types of employment the risk of unpredictable human failure is such that an artibrary retirement age is justified for application to all employees. The leading Canadian case on this defence is one decided by the Supreme Court of Canada, *Ontario Human Rights Commission* v. *Borough of Etobicoke*.[25]

Two firefighters employed by the Borough were compulsorily retired at the age of sixty according to the terms of a collective agreement. They filed a complaint under the Ontario Human Rights Code, which, like most provincial statues, including the B.C. Code, generally protects employees under the age of sixty-five. The Borough argued that the rule requiring a firefighter to retire at sixty was a bona fide occupational requirement. The Board of Inquiry held that the Borough had not proved this. The Borough appealed, and won, in an Ontario Divisional Court and the Ontario Court of Appeal.

However, the Supreme Court of Canada ruled in favour of the firefighters and restored the original decision. The Supreme Court held that the employers had the burden of proving that the rule requiring compulsory retirement was a bona fide occupational qualification, and that to establish the defence the employer must show: (1) that the limitation is imposed "honestly, in good faith, and in the sincerely held belief that such limitation is imposed in the interest of the adequate performance of the work involved with all reasonable dispatch, safety and economy and not for ulterior or extraneous reasons,"[26] and (2) that the limitation is "related in an objective sense to the performance of the employment concerned, in that it is reasonably necessary to assure the efficient and economical performance of the job without endangering the employee, his fellow employees and the general public."[27] In that case the Supreme Court held that the evidence did not establish that retirement at sixty was a bona fide occupational requirement. But in another case, *Manitoba Human Rights Commission* v. *Finalyson,*[28] a Manitoba court held that a rule requiring an active police officer to retire at sixty was permissible because of the mental and physical demands of the job.

Of course it is always open to an employer to show that an employee is no longer capable of performing his job. In the *Etobicoke* case the Court said:

> We all age chronologically at the same rate but aging in what has been termed the functional sense proceeds at widely varying rates and is largely unpredictable. In cases where concern for the employee's capacity is largely economic, that is, where the employer's concern is one of productivity and the circumstances of employment require no special skills that may diminish with aging, or involve any unusual dangers to employees or the public, it may be difficult, if not impossible, to demonstrate that a mandatory retirement at a fixed age, without regard to individual capacity, may be validly imposed under the code. In such employment, as capacity fails, and as such failure becomes evident, individuals may be discharged or retired for cause.[29]

It must be emphasized, however, that most provincial human rights legislation protects employees only until they reach the age of sixty-five. And the early decisions on section 15 of the Charter suggest that it will not affect non-governmental compulsory retirement schemes. If there is to be a change in Canadian law governing mandatory retirement, additional legislation, similar to the Age Discrimination in Employment Act in the United States, is required.

EFFECTS OF ABOLISHING MANDATORY RETIREMENT

If Canada abolished compulsory retirement, what would happen? In two recent Canadian cases[30] the arguments of the employers summarized the perceived advantages of a mandatory retirement policy, including the creation of opportunities for younger employees and the elimination of the need to make individual decisions about particular employees. These arguments deserve consideration but it must be remembered that they were prepared for partisan purposes – to convince a court that the retirement policy did not offend the Charter. American experience under the Age Discrimination in Employment Act and two major studies, one Canadian[31] and one American,[32] suggest that the abolition of mandatory retirement would have relatively little impact on our society as a whole. It might of course be very important to some individuals.

The major Canadian study is the *Report of the Commission on Compulsory Retirement* (Manitoba 1982). Among the conclusions reached in that report were the following:

(1) A relatively small percentage of the labour force would wish to continue working beyond sixty-five.[33]

(2) Because the numbers were small and their additional working years limited, they would not significantly affect youth unemployment.[34]

(3) Firms would have an incentive to introduce more effective performance appraisal systems. However, the Commission noted that this was to some extent an independent issue. Compulsory retirement is not a substitute for a performance appraisal system, and an inadequate performance appraisal system does not justify compulsory retirement.[35]

(4) Abolition of compulsory retirement would not have a material effect on government transfer payments.[36] This assumed a slight reduction in pension costs but a slight increase in youth unemployment and welfare costs.

(5) Those who continued to work would not significantly improve their post-retirement income. Concerns about inadequate pensions would be better addressed through pension reform.[37]

INCOME SECURITY AND RETIREMENT

It is difficult to conceive of the development of retirement as a common, often mandatory, social practice without the development of some scheme to provide for the future needs of those retired. Yet that was the prospect that faced many employees in the late nineteenth century. An increasing percentage of workers were employed by large industrial corporations rather than in small businesses or farming. And large corporations were concerned with the efficiency of older workers. In the words of Graebner: "Retirement to the family farm was one thing; retirement to a New York City tenement another. . . Corporate and government bureaucracies became holding institutions – informal retirement mechanisms – for thousands of older workers."[38]

Pension arrangements for particular employees are not a new idea. But it was not until the nineteenth century that North America saw the development of systematic pension plans in the modern sense. Private pension plans were developed as a technique for minimizing labour turnover. They were subject to significant restrictions and covered a small percentage of the population. Public pension schemes were introduced into Canada in 1927 (the Old Age Pension Act) and the United States in 1935 (the Social Security Act). Older persons in Canada are now eligible to receive pensions from the following public sources: (1) Old Age Security pension (OAS), (2) Guaranteed Income Supplement (GIS), and the (3) Canada/Quebec Pension Plan (C/QPPP).

What is the relative importance of public and private pension plans? From what sources do retired people derive their income?

In the *Fact Book on Aging in Canada*[39] prepared by the Government of Canada for the 1983 Conference on Aging, it was stated that in 1981 elderly married couples derived the following percentages of their income from the respective sources: OAS/GIS, 30%; C/QPP, 10%; investments, 28%; private pension plans, 13%; earnings and other, 18%. Unattached males derived somewhat more from public pension plans (43%) and private pension plans (16%). Their earnings and other income were lower (13%). Unattached females were much more dependent on public pension plans (50%) and they received less income from private pension plans (7%) or from earnings and other income (10%).[40] It should be emphasized that for all three groups, public pension plans were significantly more important than private pension plans. Within the public pension plans, the percentage derived from the C/QPP was steadily increasing.

This mix of private/public pension funds has been the subject of numerous reports and discussions, culminating in the *Report of the Parliamentary Task Force*[41] submitted in December 1983, and the partial implementation of its proposals in the May 1985 budget proposals of the Minister of Finance. This debate took place against the background of a report from the National Council on Welfare[42] on the incomes of the aged, which concluded that: (1) one aged Canadian in four lives below the poverty line; and (2) although only 11.7 per cent of families with elderly heads had incomes below the low-income line, 60 per cent of unattached elderly women and 49 per cent of unattached elderly men lived below that line.

Private pension plans have been criticized because: (1) only a minority of employees are covered; (2) the vesting of interests may be unduly delayed; (3) employees may lose accumulated pension rights if they change employment; and (4) spouses – usually women – were often left with no retirement income in the event of the death of the employee or marriage breakdown. Moreover, the tax incentives for private pension plans create a whole new range of ethical issues. In a period of financial restraint, how can incentives that generally favour the rich in our community be justified?

Faced with these realities the Canadian government had two main options: (1) improve the public pension plans to ensure that every aged person has an adequate income; or (2) encourage the development of better private pension plans *and* improve the public pension plans to ensure that the minimum needs of every aged person are met.

The government has selected the second option. In his May 1985 budget proposals, the Minister of Finance in the recently elected Progressive Conservative government moved to improve private pension schemes by amendments to the Pension Benefits Standards Act. The previous Liberal government had increased the GIS by $50 – a clear indication that the public pension schemes are to be retained as a safety net to meet minimum needs.

Some comments should be made about this decision. First, major changes in the C/QPP require the approval of two-thirds of the included provinces having at least two-thirds of the population covered by the Plan. Had the federal government proposed major changes to the C/QPP, it is not certain that it would have received the provinces' consent. However, the federal Pension Benefits Standards Act affects only some 600 employer-sponsored plans. There are some 14,000 employer-sponsored plans regulated by provincial legislation. Most provinces have, or are planning, new legislation governing private pensions. At one stage it appeared that the legislation would follow a common model. It now appears, however, that there will be significant differences in the provincial legislation.

Many feel that the federal government's actions have been too timid. In the debate on the February 1984 Liberal government budget, the Honourable Monique Bégin, then Minister of National Health and Welfare, said: "The private sector is getting one more chance with those good tax offers. They can start developing plans for their employees, particularly those in small business. Otherwise it will have to be mandatory for all Canadians, of course with the agreement of the provinces which have the jurisdiction."[43] Why was the government so timid? Clearly it was concerned about imposing additional costs on a fragile economy. The Honourable Monique Bégin said: "We could have been bolder, but as Canadians agree we should try to develop jobs first and then slowly build in good pensions for the future."[44]

Similar views have been expressed by the Honourable Jake Epp, Minister of National Health and Welfare in the Progressive Conservative government. He commented: "For too long, I believe, economic policy and social policy have been treated in isolation. . . Canadians are not prepared to see a greater and greater percentage of our finances devoted to carrying interest charges on the national debt when our social services and hospitals are choked for funds, yet that is exactly what was threatened."[45] The inference was clear. Major changes in social programs would have to be postponed until the federal deficit was reduced. On the other hand, Mr. Epp welcomed the pension reforms effected by the changes to the Pension Benefits Standards Act and the Canada Pension Plan because "more Canadians will be able to contemplate a secure and rewarding retirement if they have planned previously in their working life for their retirement."[46]

What are the ethical issues here? The current position is consistent with an ethical position that leaves each individual free to make his or her own arrangements for future income security – with society's responsibility limited to ensuring that the minimal needs of each aged individual are met. The overwhelming evidence is that this system has left a substantial number of single individuals in poverty. The alternative is to reorganize the economic resources of society to provide everyone with a good pension.

It might be argued that this is not an ethical question, that the decision is merely a practical judgment based on economic considerations. The reality is that many statements that purport to be based on economic considerations conceal ethical judgments. The state *could* provide more generous benefits – by reallocating funds from health or defence or by raising taxes. The ethical issue is how far the state should go in redistributing wealth. In a report on pension reform,[47] the National Council on Welfare acknowledged the apparent victory of the regulatory approach to pension reform but argued that "expanding the Canada and Quebec Pension Plans is the only way to ensure an adequate retirement income for Canadians who earn average wages or less during their working years."[48]

FUNDING INCOME SECURITY FOR THE ELDERLY

In the real world there is no horn of plenty. The rights of elderly Canadians to adequate income security cannot be considered in isolation from the obligations and ability to pay of the working population. The Old Age Security pension (OAS) and the income-tested Guaranteed Income Supplement (GIS) are paid out of general taxation revenues. Many people think that the Canada and Quebec Pension Plans (C/QPP) are funded programmes similar to many private schemes. In fact the C/QPP is largely funded on a pay-as-you-go basis and the Parliamentary Task Force on Pension Reform recommended no change in this basic procedure: "The Task Force recommends that the Canada and Quebec Pension Plans be funded on a pay-as-you-go basis. Calculation of the contribution rate should provide for a contingency reserve equal to 2 or 3 years' anticipated payout. It should also accommodate potential economic fluctuations and demographic situations. There should also be no sharp jumps in contribution rates from one year to the next."[49]

Even without improvements in the C/QPP, it is estimated that contributions will have to rise from the current 3.8 per cent to the 10–12.5 per cent range by 2030. Improvements advocated by the National Council on Welfare would require contributions of approximately 21 per cent by that year.[50] Whether changed or not, our income-security system for the aged involves an intergenerational transfer of wealth from the younger, working segment of the population to the older, retired segment. When we plan for our future retirement we are expecting our children to be more generous to us than we have been to our parents' generation. The extent of this intergenerational transfer is somewhat concealed. Contributors to the C/QPP are encouraged to think of it as if it were a funded insurance scheme. It is described in government publications as a "compulsory contributory earnings-related" plan. In a discussion of the comparable U.S. Social Security system, one American writer, Robinson Hollister, has talked about the "myth" of social security and speculated that the myth may be necessary to maintain the political viability of the social security programme: "A system which explicitly recognizes the separate functions of the current system – shifting funds from earnings to later life on the one hand and income maintenance on the other – will be socially divisive. The system must be shrouded in the social myth of contributory social insurance in order to operate."[51] And: "Is the social myth a necessity?. . . What is necessary to avoid conflict between the young and the old or the rich and the poor? Must we have the confidence man in order to build social institutions? While I would like to think not, I cannot argue the point with much persuasion."[52]

It may be argued that in Canada these criticisms are not valid because we distinguish between the GIS and the C/QPP. There is some validity in this comment, but there is a hope and expectation that the development of the C/QPP will reduce the need for the GIS.

The method of funding the C/QPP does raise some ethical issues. Because it is presented as a "contributory, earnings-related" plan, a significant burden is borne by those at the lower income levels. In comparison with the taxation system, it is regressive rather than progressive. Moreover, the potential for generational conflict will increase in the next century. Leroy Stone and Michael MacLean have predicted that there may be a slight increase in the percentage of government revenues required for senior citizen transfer payments between now and 2001.

> However, as the baby boom starts to dominate (numerically) the ranks of senior citizens, in the opening decades of the next century, there will be substantial pressure to add another three percentage point share of public revenues to senior citizen transfer payments. This addition does not look very large in itself; but in the context of heavy competition among alternative programs for relatively scarce public revenues the pressure to add those percentage points could lead to significant political and economic difficulties.[53]

What, you may ask, are the ethical issues involved in funding income security for the elderly? To return to my original theme, it is a question of how far the individual's right to the product of his labour is to be qualified in order to ensure desired social goals. This particular ethical issue would not arise if the C/QPP were a fully funded plan. What would remain as an ethical issue is the allocation of responsibility between the individual and the state for planning for the individual's future income security. There are strong practical reasons for expanding the C/QPP. But that involves a surrender of personal autonomy.

It is not surprising that the concept of compulsory retirement is under attack in Canada. It is a concept that has outlived its usefulness. Nor is it surprising that there is so much controversy over pension policy. But the ethical issues are confused – by the myths surrounding the C/QPP and economic judgments that conceal the underlying issues. The pressures that will develop in the next thirty to forty years may expose the underlying ethical issues – and the complacency into which many of us have drifted.

NOTES

1 J. Bentham (1789), *An Introduction to the Principles of Morals and Legislation* in the *Works of Jeremy Bentham,* ed. by John Bowring. (New York: Russell and Russell 1962) 1:44
2 H.L.A. Hart, "Law in the Perspective of Philosophy: 1776–1976," *New York University Law Review* (1976) 51: 538–51, at 541
3 J. Rawls, *A Theory of Justice* (Cambridge, MA: Belknap Press of Harvard University Press 1971)
4 R. Nozick, *Anarchy, State and Utopia* (New York: Basic Books 1974)
5 *Op. cit. supra,* n. 3 at 302
6 *Report of the Commission on Compulsory Retirement* (Manitoba 1982), 170
7 *Report of the Parliamentary Committee on Equality Rights* (1985), 21
8 Canadian Charter of Rights and Freedoms (Part 1, Schedule B of the Constitution Act 1982), section 15
9 (1986), 30 DLR (4th) 700; [1986] 6 WWR 23 (BCSC)
10 *Harrison* v. *University of British Columbia* (1986), 30 DLR (4th) 206; [1986] 6 WWR 7 (BCSC): *Re McKinney and the University of Guelph* (1986), 32 DLR (4th) 65 (Ont. HC); *Ontario English Catholic Teachers Association* v *School Board (Roman Catholic Separate) of Essex County* (1987), 18 OAC 271 (Ont. Div. Ct.)
11 (1986), 32 DLR (4th) 65 (Ont. HC)
12 Ibid., 103
13 This figure is based on the *Report of the Commission on Compulsory Retirement* (Manitoba 1982) 185–88. The compilation of statistics from larger firms results in some overstatement of the numbers affected by compulsory retirement. In *Re McKinney and the University of Guelph* (1986), 32 DLR (4th) 65, Professors Gunderson and Pesando, economics professors at the University of Toronto, testified that approximately half of the work force in Canada are in jobs with mandatory retirement provisions (at 101).
14 William Graebner, *A History of Retirement* (New Haven: Yale University Press 1980)
15 See the studies cited in ibid., 39–40
16 Ibid., 251
17 Ibid., 215
18 W. Andrew Achenbaum, Shades of Gray: Old Age, American Values and Federal

Policies since 1920 (Boston: Little, Brown 1983), 58–62
19 *McIntire* v. *University of Manitoba* (1981), 119 DLR (3d) 252 (Man. CA)
20 *Newport* v. *Government of Manitoba* (1981), 131 DLR (3d) 564 (Man. CA)
21 *Parkinson* v. *Health Sciences Centre* (1981), 131 DLR (3d) 513 (Man. CA)
22 *Paterson* v. *E.H. Price Ltd.* (1982), 3 Can. HRRD/904
23 *Craton* v. *Winnipeg School Board* (1983), 149 DLR (3d) 542 (Man. CA); *Re Winnipeg School Division No. 1 and Craton* (1985), 21 DLR (4th) 1 (SCC)
24 The language of the statues differs. For a more detached discussion, see Elizabeth Atcheson and Lynne Sullivan, "Passage to Retirement: Age Discrimination and the Charter" in Anne Bayefsky and Mary Eberts (eds.), *Equality Rights and the Canadian Charter of Rights and Freedoms* (Toronto: Carswell 1982) 231–92, especially 251–65.
25 (1982), 132 DLR (3d) 14 (SCC)
26 Ibid., 19–20
27 Ibid., 20
28 [1983] 3 WWR 117 (Man. CA)
29 *Supra,* n. 23, at 20
30 *Re McKinney and the University of Guelph* (1986), 32 DLR (4th) 65 at 93 (Ont. HC) and *Ontario English Catholic Teachers Association* v. *School Board (Roman Catholic Separate) of Essex County* (1987), 18 OAC 271 at 276–79 (Ont. Div. Ct.)
31 *Report of the Commission on Compulsory Retirement* (Manitoba 1982)
32 *Abolishing Mandatory Retirement,* a report prepared by the U.S. Department of Labor (Washington, DC: Supt. of Docs. 1981)
33 (1985), 21 DLR (4th) 1 at 15
34 Ibid., 19
35 Ibid., 20
36 Ibid., 23
37 Ibid., 22
38 *Op. cit. supra,* n. 14 at 14
39 *Fact Book on Aging in Canada* (Ottawa: Minister of Supply and Services 1983)
40 Ibid., 46–47
41 *Report of the Parliamentary Task Force on Pension Reform* (Ottawa: House of Commons 1983)
42 *Sixty-five and Older,* a report of the National Council on Welfare (Ottawa: Minister of Supply and Services 1984)
43 *Debates,* House of Commons (Canada), 2nd Session, 32nd Parliament (1984) 2: 1567
44 Ibid., 1566
45 *Debates,* House of Commons (Canada), 1st Session, 33rd Parliament (1985) 4: 5075
46 Ibid., 5076
47 *Pension Reform,* a report of the National Council on Welfare (Ottawa: Minister of Supply and Services 1984)
48 Ibid., 44
49 *Op. cit. supra,* n. 39 at 41
50 *Op. cit. supra,* n. 47 at 50
51 Robinson Hollister "Social Mythology and Reform: Income Maintenance for the Aged" in Political Consequences of Aging, *Annals of the American Academy of Political and Social Science* (1974) 415: 19–40, at 38
52 Ibid., 39
53 Leroy O. Stone and Michael J. MacLean, *Future Income Prospects for Canada's Senior Citizens* (Montreal- Institute for Research on Public Policy 1979), 89

10

Society and Essentials for Well-Being: Social Policy and the Provision of Care

NEENA L. CHAPPELL

This paper has been written from the perspective of a sociologist, not a philosopher or an ethicist.[1] Nevertheless, ethics and morality are relevant to a social perspective. Ultimately, we are interested in a just society, one that allows for dignity and autonomy during old age. Ethical issues are those against which we assess whether our provision of care is adequate or not.

There are three sections below. The first deals with the development of the existing formal care system within Canadian society. The second presents a critique of that system. The final section presents an alternative system which, it is argued, is more likely to provide dignity, autonomy, and freedom of choice for the individual than the existing system.

DEVELOPMENT OF THE HEALTH CARE SYSTEM

It was only in the twentieth century that social security developed in a significant way in Canada, that social security legislation resulted in a clear-cut chronological age around which a social definition of old age has evolved.

During the 1920s, after the First World War, social security and specifically old age pensions became a political issue (Bryden, 1974: 75–76; Cassidy, 1943: 22). Both mothers' allowances and old age pensions were passed in Canada in this decade. The 1927 act established a national, non-contributory, means-tested pension plan at age seventy. This federal Old Age Pensions Act also established the principle of public responsibility for ensuring that the aged receive a basic subsistence allowance. It represented the first major federal intervention in the country in the social welfare field. It did so within the principle of federal-provincial cost sharing, national program standards, and provincial administration of old age pensions (Chappell 1980, 1987; Wilson 1982). The federal-provincial divisions of authority and the decentralized governmental system in this country are reflected in these principles and contrast with the centralized system found in other places, such as Great Britain.

The Depression demonstrated the social nature of human need (Irving 1980). Bryden (1974: 75–76) notes that poverty among the aged was so acute, widespread, and chronic during the 1920s that it simply could not be ignored. The aged, in fact, were not singled out as a group prior to the Second World War except for the old age assistance legislation of 1927. In the 1930s, the federal share of old age pensions increased to 75 per cent because some of the poorer provinces could not pay (Bryden 1974: 17). It was not until 1951 that an amendment to the BNA Act resulted in old age security payments to all persons aged seventy and over, irrespective of means, later lowered to age sixty-five.

Canadian policy has been described as evolving in a continuous process of experimentation (Leman 1977). Canada has built a successive policy of social security that is constantly undergoing change and redefinition. It began in 1927. In 1951 the original act was replaced with the Old Age Security Act, giving a universal flat pension to all those seventy and over, and the Old Age Assistance Act, which provided means-tested old age assistance starting at age sixty-five. In 1965 the development of contributory social insurance was matched with income-tested supplementation.

The involvement of the national government in the area of health service legislation occurred after the development of income security legislation. Prior to this, however, governments were already involved in some areas related to health. For example, in the early part of the century, there was government involvement with workmen's compensation medical services; municipal doctors on salary in Saskatchewan and Alberta; hospital outpatient departments for the indigent and near-indigent; public clinics for VD, TB, child welfare, and so on; federal medical services for war veterans; and health plans operated by numerous industries. Public effort was most effective in the area of public health or preventive medicine, such as in the collection of vital statistics, sanitary inspection, supervision of water, milk, and food, and the like.

In addition, the beginning of public acceptance of medicine is usually placed around the late 1800s and early 1900s (Brown 1979; Coburn et al. 1981; Enos & Sultan 1977: 188–96). Early in the seventeenth century, William Harvey discovered the circulation of blood; in the late nineteenth century, Pasteur discovered that each disease had its own causative microorganism and Lister advanced techniques for sterilizing surgical procedures. It was also in the late nineteenth century that a vaccine for smallpox was found, and the stethoscope, clinical thermometer, and hypodermic syringe were invented (Enos & Sultan 1977: 188–96). The first two decades of the twentieth century saw the passage of medical licensing laws, standardization of medical schools, restrictions on entry into the medical field, and increases in the income and status of the medical profession.

Cassidy (1943: 23) informs us that it was in the 1930s, during the Depression, when a great interest in health insurance developed in Canada. This was the decade after old age pension legislation had been passed and a time when private enterprise dominated the field of health. Doctors, dentists, and nurses sold their services privately. Drugs and medicines were sold on the market. Before the federal government assumed welfare functions previously considered the responsibility of the provinces, thousands of individuals could not afford care. The lack of standardization of services from one local area to another and the lack of central co-ordination became evident. Social services were unable to meet the growing demand (Bryden, 1974: 14–21).

In 1940, Prime Minister William Lyon Mackenzie King requested the Rowell-Sirois Commission to study the economic problems of Canada and the nature of federal-provincial relations. A Committee on Reconstruction was established in 1941, with Leonard Marsh appointed Research Director. Marsh was a British-born economist who had worked for Beverage at the London School of Economics. In 1942, two weeks after the release of the Beverage Report in England, the Committee began work on the report on social security for Canada, the Marsh Report. Marsh argued that if social security was to be basically sound, it would have to be underwritten by the community as a whole for the universal risks of sickness and invalidity in old age. The first suggestion was for a national health insurance scheme.

Implementation began in 1945 with half of Marsh's main points. Both a research and training program and assistance in hospital construction were put into place (Marsh 1975: xxii). The Hospital Insurance and Diagnostic Services Act of 1957 ensured hospital care for the entire population through a fiscal policy in which the federal government agreed to share the cost of running hospitals (excluding special institutions). In 1960, the Guaranteed Income Supplement Program gave additional funds to old age pensioners whose incomes fell below a certain level. In 1964 old age pensions were extended to include income-tested supplements, including survivor's disability benefits irrespective of age. In 1965–66, the Medical Care Act was passed (although it was not implemented until 1968), providing a national insurance scheme for physician services, and the 1966 Canada Assistance Plan provided social assistance to anyone in need. This plan, however, was means-tested and varied from province to province. Also in 1966, the Canada/Quebec Pension Plan came into being, and after a ten-year transition period it became fully effective (Bryden 1974: 8, 104, 125; Collins 1978: 112,

117; Government of Canada 1970: 8, 94; LeClair 1975; Lee 1974).

All provinces and territories had joined the federal government's cost-shared comprehensive medical insurance program by 1972. Eligibility criteria included universal coverage, reasonable access to services, portability of benefits, comprehensive services, and non-profit administration by a public agency. Prior to 1977, federal-provincial cost sharing was fifty-fifty, with the federal government matching every dollar a province spent on approved services.

In 1977 this was changed to a system of cash grants from federal to the provincial governments based on population, gross national product, and the transfer of specific taxing powers to the provinces. Because the funds were divorced from specific health expenditures, the rate of growth of federal costs was limited. The provinces also had more control over specific health expenditures within their own territory, since transfers were no longer dependent on the use of specified services.

The federal government passed the Canada Health Act of 1984 because of concern over a threat to reasonable access. This arose because of the increase in extra-billing by physicians (additional charges to patients over and above the payment schedule), and hospital user fees within provinces to help finance their share of health insurance costs. This Act provides for a reduction in federal financial contributions to provincial health plans by the amount of extra-billing and user charges implemented in the provinces.

The social security program in Canada began health coverage with the provision of medical services, hospital services, and physician services. It now provides a mix of federal and provincial programs focusing on the income and health areas. Medical services and some social services are provided.

THE RESULTANT HEALTH CARE SYSTEM

A striking feature of Canada's health care system is its focus on medical care. Even though only about 19 per cent of total health care expenditures go directly to physicians, this group largely controls hospital utilization, prescription of drugs, and so forth (Bennett & Krasny 1981; Detsky 1978). Evans (1976, 1984) estimates that physicians, as the main gatekeepers of the system, control 80 per cent of health care costs. The decision to use expensive health services is not made by the individual patient or client, but primarily by medical doctors. Further, a third-party insurance system does nothing to encourage cost-effective utilization. It pays physicians on a fee for service basis (Bird & Fraser 1981). In addition, while hospital space and resources have been more or less stable since the 1970s, the number of physicians has continued to grow. This has resulted in increased pressure for hospital capacity (Evans 1984: 176).

The medical orientation has also led to a growth in the use of drugs and medication, particularly with the development of sulpha and antibiotic drugs which were effective against diseases such as pneumonia and bacterial infections. This growth is evident among the population as a whole, but especially so among elderly individuals (Chappell & Barnes 1982). Although elderly individuals constitute about 10 per cent of the population in the United States, they received approximately 25 per cent of all prescriptions written in 1967. In that same year, persons over sixty-five required roughly three times as many prescribed drugs and spent more than three times as much for their drugs than did those under that age (Peterson 1978). As a group, elderly persons are the largest consumers of legal drugs and are increasing the number of prescriptions purchased annually (Guttman 1978; Chappell et al. 1986).

Together with the emphasis on physician services and treatment with drugs, there has also developed an institutional bias within the health care system. The development of medicine as a profession has been tied intimately to the development of short-term institutional services, specifically with hospitals. In Canada, it was after the Second World War that hospitals developed and signalled a break with home care, which had traditionally been how illness was treated. By this time hospitals were viewed as a place where skilled medical specialists practised and complex diagnostic technologies were utilized (Coburn et al. 1983).

As noted earlier, hospital growth was federally supported in the 1940s and 1950s through contributions towards their construction. The growth of hospitals encouraged the development of hospital insurance, since hospitalization expenses could be very high. This became confounded with the addition of medical insurance, because the growth of hospitals resulted in physicians becoming increasingly specialized, hospital-minded, and used to expensive therapies (Tsalikis 1982). It also resulted in the growth of paramedical workers to assist in the tasks performed within this setting. Indeed, the hospital has been considered the major factor in transforming the work of doctors from independent entrepreneurship to a complex medical-industrial institution.

The focus on hospitals reinforces short-term acute care. Care for elderly persons, essentially chronic care, has been provided through long-term care institutions, variously referred to as nursing homes, personal care homes, and so on, where the focus is custodial (Eisdorfer & Cohen 1982: 82–88).

Perhaps most dramatically illustrating our emphasis on physician and institutional services and the concomitant lack of emphasis on home care services are the proportions of total expenditures within the system. In Canada, for the period from 1970 to 1979, 50 per cent of total health care expenditures went to hospitals and nursing homes, that it, institutional care; 25 per cent went to salaries for professional services, including but not limited to physician services; 10 per cent went to drugs and appliances; and 15 per cent to all other costs (Statistics Canada 1983: 9)

Not until the 1970s was there noticeable growth in home health services. At that time a broad definition of services evolved and home care started to be viewed as a service in its own right. However, the lack of national co-ordination and Canada's decentralized system makes it difficult to compile even basic statistics in this area. Currently, a lack of uniformity from province to province characterizes programme objectives, criteria, funding sources, services available, personnel, and terminology (Government of Canada 1982).

The focus on physician-centred services and institutional care has resulted in the acceptance of a medical model of health and illness. Indeed there is a tendency in society to equate good health with proper medical care and to identify health with medicine. This implies that an extension and expansion of health care services would be accompanied by rises in health levels within the population (Mishler 1981a).

A medical focus assumes by and large a biomedical model of health and illness. This perspective assumes that etiology is biologically specific, that is, disease is accounted for by deviations from the norm of measurable biological variables. Medical care and treatment are defined primarily as technical problems whereby the goals of medicine are viewed in terms of technical criteria such as validity, diagnosis, provision of disease-related treatment, symptom relief, and termination of disease processes. This is reinforced by the training done in large teaching hospitals filled with large-scale medical technology (Mishler 1981b, c).

This biomedical perspective has resulted in a focus on cure and acute care rather than chronic illness and coping with permanent conditions. Indeed, some argue it has resulted in old age itself being defined as a problem considered solvable through the receipt of services, essentially medical services, at the individual level (Estes 1979).

Recently, criticisms of the biomedical model have been rampant. Indeed, a physician friend says that "physician bashing" has become a national pastime. The remainder of this paper is not intended in any way as a derogation of individual physicians. Many, and perhaps most, are hardworking, committed individuals. It is, however, intended as a criticism of the entire system and a plea for a restructuring and reorganization of that system to better meet the needs of an aging society.

One of the main criticisms of the medical model is that it does not take into account socially defined meaning. Even when defining a biological norm or deviation, one must take into account specific populations and their sociocultural characteristics in order to be accurate (Mishler 1981b). It is further argued that physicians do not simply apply technical knowledge but also impart social messages. The structure within which medical services are delivered, including the doctor-patient relationship, is social in nature. These relationships reflect the social relationships of the larger society with their class, race, sex, and age differences (J. Ehrenreich 1975; B. Ehrenreich, 1978; Estes 1979). A prime example cited by these authors is the treatment of menstruation and pregnancy in the latter part of the nineteenth century. Both were considered signs of illness and treated with rest and passivity. Indeed, this "illness" was used as a reason for excluding women from paid labour. That is, the diagnosis and treatment reflected the male dominance of the society.

In relation to aging, it is argued that the medical profession promotes and also reflects the belief that elderly individuals are in need of services, in particular health services which are equated with medical services. By and large, national health policies are remedial and do not address the disadvantaged status of aging individuals and the need to improve their social and economic status.

These attacks on the medical profession come at a time when a powerful, expensive, and complex industrial-pharmaceutical-medical system is firmly in place. The basic system has not undergone major transformation despite the fact that McKeown (McKeown & Lowe 1966; McKeown et al. 1975), Dubos (1963) and McKinlay and McKinlay (1977) have shown that medical intervention was not the primary cause of declines in mortality in this century. Maxwell (1975) and Weller and Manga (1982) have shown that the major diseases of old age are chronic and not acute, and health care expenditures are not necessarily correlated with health outcomes. Syme and Berkman (1981) and Grant (1984) have shown that social class and poverty are significantly correlated with health.

In addition, attempts have been made to relate cost figures and concomitantly number of physicians with health outcomes. Both developed and less developed countries show a high correlation between life expectancy and number of physicians, up to a level of 100 physicians per 100,000 population. After that point the relationship is not clear. Canada's health expenditures are higher than Great Britain's but Canada has a lower life expectancy. Similarly, the United States spends a higher proportion of GNP on health care than any other country in the world, but has the next to worst mortality rate among Western nations (Bennett & Krasny 1981; Maxwell 1975).

It is also clear that the nature of illness has shifted. Infectious diseases have been replaced as major causes of death by heart disease, cancer, and other chronic illnesses, as well as accidents and other conditions related to life style. More dollars spent on the current medical care system are unlikely to yield freedom from these illnesses. Further, the major illnesses of old age are chronic in nature, or are acute episodes of chronic illnesses. The most frequent chronic conditions are heart disease, arthritis, chronic rheumatism, and hypertension (Neugarten 1982). Thus, the elderly need services to help them cope with chronic conditions and functional disability.

Other critics present more extreme arguments: not only is medicine not responsible for many of the improvements in life and health, but modern scientific medicine has had a negative impact on health. Perhaps best known in this regard is Illich (1977) and his concept of iatrogenesis. Iatrogenesis refers to diseases and other individual and social problems resulting from the practice of medicine itself. Examples include side-effects and addictions associated with drugs, unnecessary surgery, accidents, and injuries and infections resulting from hospitalization. Illich argues further that the intrusion of the medical definition into more and more aspects of life erodes individual autonomy for self-care and community processes for mutual care. Individuals become less and less competent to take care of themselves.

The critique continues. Others, such as Friedson (1963, 1970a, b), have argued that physicians, in fact, are great imperialsists. Friedson maintains that the demand for a monopoly control of the profession by the profession may have less to do with the corpus of specialized and technical knowledge of medicine which is used to justify this demand than with efforts to sustain the position of power and status of physicians vis-à-vis other health professionals and vis-à-vis their patients.

The power of the medical profession is evident in its official role at birth, at death, and in between. Increasingly, areas previously outside the jurisdiction of medicine are coming under its aegis – alcoholism and other addictions are viewed as illnesses; mental illness is considered a disease; death and dying now take place in the hospital. Physicians make critical decisions relating to workmen's compensation and mothers' allowances, and play other certifying roles. They are well represented on critical policy and planning committees throughout society. They are heavily involved in research, not to mention their more obvious roles as educators of future physicians and certifiers of illness.

As expressed so adequately by Mishler (1981a, b, c), the criticisms of the biomedical approach are not simply an argument to incorporate epidemiological or other social variables in the consideration of the biological. Nor are they simply an argument that one should be aware of the effects of medical practice and institutional and organizational factors on the practice of medicine. Whenever it is argued that meaning is socially constructed, the meaning of health and illness is included. This leads one to view diagnosis as interpretive work, that is, as one of several ways through which reality is viewed. Some argue further that medicine is not only social practice, but that this practice has functional significance for the larger society. That is, the health care system in Canada is to a considerable extent centralized around a medical model of health and illness, and in particular around the services of physicians and around both acute and long-term institutional care. These emphases are critical in assessing the adequacy of the health care system for an aging society.

AN ALTERNATIVE HEALTH CARE SYSTEM

If the social meaning and consequences of the biomedical model are not fully understood, the emphasis on technical expertise and bioscientific knowledge to improve levels of health will be considered appropriate by policy planners, medical educators, and health administrators. Energy and funding will be directed to improving the existing system, such as ensuring a more equitable distribution of physicians or more effective application of scientific medicine. As long as it is assumed that the basic premises underlying the system are correct, the current policies are not questioned and more resources are put into improving the existing system.

As Crichton (1980) notes, one can spend endless efforts increasing access to the current system, or increasing patient satisfaction and distribution of physicians or increasing utilization of hospital beds, but if these do not have much bearing on health outcome, the effort is not going to achieve its goal. Issues of health education, preventive measures, environmental health, and health promotion are all relatively neglected within the current system.

In looking at an alternative health care system, the underlying principles of universality and equal access should not be compromised. Further, an alternative health care system would include the medical profession and a medical perspective as a legitimate part, but with considerably less dominance than is evident today. It would include a greater emphasis on individual patient autonomy, the inclusion of the informal network in the care of elderly people, and social and community services. Programs should be developed which allow a flexibility of relationships between caregivers, whether professional or non-professional, over a long period of time. This assumes that the significance of chronic disease be measured in terms of the extent to which an individual's ability to function is impaired, and that the satisfactory care of the chronically ill include many aspects, such as income, housing, and social support (Vladeck & Firman 1983).

There has to be a greater emphasis on chronic care, specifically chronic home care; a greater emphasis on meeting the needs of the patient, including a recognition of the potential for rehabilitation among elderly persons, rather than an emphasis on only custodial care; and a greater emphasis on flexibility within the system, especially long-term institutional care, so that individuals can and will return to the community.

All of this assumes a broad definition of health, such as the one adopted by the World Health Organization, recognizing that quality of life entails more than biomedical aspects. When health is no longer equated with medicine, health care can become associated with healing activities. A broad definition leads to activities and expenditures aimed at preserving an acceptable equilibrium between the person and his or her environment. Programs directed toward health involve strategies of public health, preventive medicine, and health maintenance. Chronic care and home care should be key words within a broad health care system

An alternative system would also assume more interfacing between the formal and informal systems of care than currently exists. Informal care also includes self-care. It is frequently forgotten that self-care, not professional care, constitutes the majority of personal health care; that people usually try to treat problems themselves prior to seeking formal medical care; and that among those who seek care and ultimately obtain a prescription, a combination of the formal remedy and their own often exists (DeFriese & Woomert 1983). The majority of elderly persons are capable of caring – and do care – for themselves on a day-to-day basis.

The informal care system, including family, friends, and neighbours, is estimated to provide approximately 80 per cent of all care to elderly individuals in society (Brody 1980; Chappell 1985). That is, the current health care system provides only about 20 per cent of all care. A reorganized formal system would ensure both flexibility and facilitation of self and informal care. An important aspect of this would be respite care for informal caregivers.

A more appropriate system demands wholesale change in the existing *medical* care system with movement towards a *health* care system. The critical issues for an aging society involve the development of a health care system and the delivery of health care services than can best improve the health status of individuals. Evans (1984) argues that major changes are possible without upheaval in the structure of society. Viewing the system as a whole can make a difference. All forms of questionable utilization should be dealt with. The change must be global, not partial. If substitutes for inpatient care are funded, corresponding components of inpatient capacity should be withdrawn.

I argued briefly here that the current formal health care system is primarily a medical care system. Such a system must be reorganized and restructured if we are to have a system which ensures individual dignity, autonomy, and freedom of choice.

NOTE

1 This is an abbreviated version of a much longer argument. More details can be found in N.L. Chappell, L.A. Strain, and A.H. Blandford, *Aging and Health Care: A Social Perspective* (Toronto: Holt, Rinehart, & Winston 1986).

REFERENCES

Bennett, J.E., & Krasny, J. (1981). Health care in Canada. In D. Coburn, C. D'Arcy, P. New, and G. Torrance (Eds.), *Health and Canadian society: Sociological perspectives*. Don Mills, Ont.: Fitzhenry & Whiteside

Bird, R.M., & Fraser, R.D. (1981). *Commentaries on the Hall Report*. Toronto: Ontario Economic Council.

Brody, E.M. (1980). Innovative programs and services for elderly and family. Testimony before the *Select Committee on Aging*, House of Representatives, 96th Congress, Washington, DC

Brown, E.R. (1979). *Rockefeller medicine men: Medicine and capitalism in America*. Berkeley, CA: University of California Press

Bryden, K. (1974). *Old age pensions and policy-making in Canada*. Montreal: McGill-Queen's University Press

Cassidy, H.M. (1943). *Social security and reconstruction*. Toronto: Ryerson

Chappell, N.L. (1980). Social policy and the elderly. In V.W. Marshall (Ed.), *Aging in Canada: Social perspectives*. Don Mills: Fitzhenry & Whiteside

Chappell, N.L. (1985). Social support and the receipt of home care services. *The Gerontologist, 25*, 47–54

Chappell, N.L. (1987). Canadian income and health-care policy: Implications for the elderly. In V.W. Marshall (Ed.), *Aging in Canada*, 2nd ed. Markham, Ont. Fitzhenry & Whiteside

Chappell, N.L., & Barnes, G.E. (1982). The practicing pharmacist and the elderly client. *Contemporary Pharmacy Practice, 5*, 170–75

Chappell, N.L., Strain, L.A., & Blandford, A.A. (1986). *Aging and health care: A social perspective*. Toronto: Holt, Rinehart, & Winston of Canada

Coburn, D., D'Arcy, C., New, P. & Torrance, G. (1981). *Health and Canadian society sociological perspectives*. Don Mills: Fitzhenry & Whiteside

Coburn, D., Torrance, G.M., & Kaufert, J.M. (1983). Medical dominance in Canada: The rise and fall of medicine. *International Journal of Health Services, 13*, 407–32

Collins, K. (1978). *Women and pensions*. Ottawa: Canadian Council on Social Development

Crichton, A. (1980). Equality: A concept in Canadian health care: From intention to reality of provision. *Social Science and Medicine, 14C*, 243–57

DeFriese, G.H., & Woomert, A. (1983). Self-care among U.S. elderly: Recent developments. *Research in Aging, 5*, 3–23

Detsky, A.S. (1978). *The economic foundations of national health policy*. Cambridge, MA: Balinger Publishing

Dubos, R.J. (1963). Infection into disease. In D.J. Ingle (Ed.), *Life and disease*. New York: Basic Books

Ehrenreich, B. (1975). The health care industry: A theory of industrial medicine. *Social Policy, 6*, 4–11

Ehrenreich, J. (Ed.) (1978). *The cultural crisis of modern medicine*. New York: Monthly Review Press

Eisdorfer, C., & Cohen, D. (1982). *Mental health care of the aging: A multidisciplinary curriculum for professional training*. New York: Springer Publishing

Enos, D.D., & Sultan, P. (1977). *The sociology of health care: Social, economic and political perspectives*. New York: Praeger Publishers

Estes, C.L. (1979). *The aging enterprise*. San Francisco: Jossey-Bass

Evans, R.G. (1976). Does Canada have too many doctors? Why nobody loves an immigrant physician. *Canadian Public Policy II*, 147–60

Evans, R.G. (1984). *Strained mercy: The economics of Canadian health care*. Toronto: Butterworths

Friedson, E. (Ed.) (1963). *The hospital in modern society*. New York: Free Press of Glencoe

Friedson, E. (1970a). *Professions of medicine: A study of the sociology of applied knowledge*. New York: Harper Row Publishers

Friedson, E. (1970b). *Professional dominance: The social structure of medical care*. New York: Atherton Press

Government of Canada. (1970). *Income security and social services: Government of Canada working paper on the constitution*. Ottawa: Queen's Printer

Government of Canada. (1982). *Canadian government report on aging*. Ottawa: Minister of Supply and Services

Grant, K.R. (1984). The inverse care law in the context of universal free health insurance in Canada: Toward meeting health needs through social policy. *Sociological Focus, 17*, 137–155

Guttman, D. (1978). Patterns of legal drug use by older Americans. *Addictive Diseases, 3*, 337

Illich, I. (1977). *The medical nemesis*. New York: Random House

Irving, A. (1980). *The development of income security in Canada, Britain and the United States, 1908–1945: A comparative and interpretive account*. (Publication Series, Working Papers on Social Welfare in Canada) Toronto: University of Toronto, Faculty of Social Work

LeClair, M. (1975). The Canadian health care system. In S. Andreopoulos (Ed.), *National health insurance: Can we learn from Canada?* New York: John Wiley & Sons

Lee, S.S. (1974). Health insurance in Canada: An overview and commentary. *New England Journal of Medicine, 290*, 713

Leman, C. (1977). Patterns of policy development: Social security in the United States and Canada. *Public Policy, 25*, 261–91

Marsh, L. (1975). *Report on social security for Canada*. Toronto: University of Toronto (reprint)

Maxwell, R. (1975). *Health care: The growing dilemma*. New York: McKinsey

McKeown, T., and Lowe, C.R. (1966). *An introduction to social medicine*. Philadelphia: F.A. Davis

McKeown, T., Record, R.G., & Turner, R.D. (1975). An interpretation of the decline of mortality in England and Wales during the twentieth century. *Population Studies, 29*, 391–422

McKinlay, J.B., & McKinlay, S.M. (1977). The questionable contribution of medical measures to the decline of mortality in the United States in the twentieth century. *Milbank Memorial Fund Quarterly, summer*

Mishler, E.G. (1981a). Social contents of health care. In E.G. Mishler, L.R. Amarasingham, S.T. Hauser, S.D. Osherson, N.E. Waxler, and R. Liem (Eds.), *Social contexts of health, illness and patient care*. Cambridge: Cambridge University Press

Mishler, E.G. (1981b). The health care system: Social contexts and consequences. In E.G. Mishler, L.R. Amarasingham, S.T. Hauser, S.D. Osherson, N.E. Waxler, and R. Liem (Eds.), *Social contexts of health, illness and patient care*. Cambridge: Cambridge University Press

Mishler, E.G. (1981c). In conclusion: A new perspective of health and medicine. In E.G. Mishler, L.R. Amarasingham, S.T. Hauser, S.D. Osherson, N.E. Waxler, and R. Liem (Eds.), *Social contexts of health, illness and patient care*. Cambridge: Cambridge University Press

Neugarten, B.L. (Ed.) (1982). Policy for the 1980's: Age or need entitlement? In *Age or need? Public policies for older people*. Beverly Hills, CA: Sage Publications
Peterson, D.M. (1983). Drug use among the aged. *Addictive Diseases, 3,* 305.
Statistics Canada. (1983). *Fact book on aging in Canada*. Ottawa: Minister of Supply and Services
Syme, S.L., & Berkman, L.F. (1981). Social class, susceptibility and sickness. In P. Conrad and R. Kern (Eds.), *The sociology of health and illness: Critical perspectives*. New York: St. Martin's Press
Tsalikis, G. (1982). Canada. In M.C. Hokenstad and R.A. Ritvo (Eds.), *Linking health care and social services*. Beverly Hills, CA: Sage Publications
Vladeck, B.C., & Firman, J.P. (1983). The aging of the population and health services. *Annals of the American Academy of Political and Social Science*, 132–48
Weller, G.R., & Manga, P. (1982). *The reprivatisation of hospital and medical care services: A comparative analysis of Canada, Britain and the United States*. Revised version of the paper presented at the *10th World Congress of Sociology*, Mexico City, November
Wilson, L. (1982). Historical perspectives: Canada. In W.M. Edwards and F. Flynn (Eds.), *Gerontology: A cross-national core list of significant works*. Ann Arbor: University of Michigan Press

11

Foregoing Treatment: Killing vs. Letting Die and the Issue of Non-feeding

EARL R. WINKLER

While the two main questions I discuss in this paper[1] are not of exclusive concern to the aged, they do concern them prominently. I will first consider the question of the moral relevance of the killing/letting die distinction. This issue is crucial in assessing the rationality of the current absolute prohibitions of direct killing in medical contexts, embodied both in law and in codes of ethics. Furthermore, this issue bears directly upon my second main question, whether the withdrawal of foods and fluids from a patient is ever morally permissible. Between the sections in which I take up these questions, I interpose some commentary on relevant parts of the United States Presidential Commission Report on *Deciding to Forego Life-Sustaining Treatment* (1983) and the Canadian Law Reform Commission Report, *Euthanasia, Aiding Suicide and Cessation of Treatment* (1983).

THE KILLING/LETTING DIE DISTINCTION

Everyone agrees that it is usually morally worse to actually kill than to merely allow death to occur. And nearly everyone agrees that there can be instances in which the two behaviours would be morally equivalent. The centre of the dispute over moral relevance concerns the reason why killing is generally worse than letting die. Does this have anything to do with what defines an act as a killing, or is this typical moral difference a result of other common associated factors, like differences in motive or intention or the certainty of the result?

Acts/omissions. It can seem that the killing/letting die distinction is essentially based on the broader distinction between acts and omissions. Roughly, one kills by actively doing something that directly causes death, whereas one allows death to occur by refraining from doing something that would have preserved life under the circumstances. At best, however, this is merely a convenient glossing over, for in some circumstances one is appropriately said to kill by refraining from some action (killing by starvation, for example) and in others one allows death to occur by doing something (issuing orders against resuscitation).

Causal instrumentality. Departing form an acts/omissions account, one naturally adopts a characterization in terms of form and degree of causal instrumentality or involvement in the death. In general, the difference between killing and letting die is a difference in the directness and prominence of an agent's causal role in the events leading to death. From this point of view, the principal argument against the moral relevance of the distinction is easily summarized. Tautologically, what centrally matters for morality is moral responsibility for death, and therefore, if the intentions, motives, and outcomes are the same between killing and permitting death to occur, it cannot make any moral difference what form of causal instrumentality is involved. That is, under these conditions both behaviours constitute the intentional termination of a life; hence moral responsibility is equivalent, and it does not matter that one behaviour employs causal means that constitute direct killing while the other exploits indirect causal means.[2] This has been a very influential position, particularly among philosophers, though it appears to have had less impact in other quarters. Most importantly, however, even those who accept this specific conclusion frequently go on to argue that, for reasons of long-term social utility related to potential abuse and misapplication, it does not follow that policies allowing killing should be permitted within medical institutions. I will later return to this point.

Normative force of the distinction. An interesting and important difficulty with this position when taken quite generally concerns the way in which normative considerations, connected with requirements, expectations, prerogatives, and powers pertaining to social and professional roles, may influence the very application of the distinction in question. Normative considerations of these kinds often have quite a determinative effect upon our understanding of an agent's causal role and involvement in a death, and hence upon the way we classify the act. For example, imagine an airplane mechanic who carefully follows all required procedures in installing a certain critical part that happens to be defective; the part fails, causing a crash that kills several people. This mechanic would not be seen as causally responsible for this event; the principal and significant cause would be located in the defective and malfunctioning part. However, causal agency and responsibility would be seen quite differently if someone who was clearly unqualified and unauthorized to perform such repairs were similarly to install a defective part with like results. While from an abstract perspective the specific actions of both agents may make the same material, causal contribution to the crash and ensuing deaths, because of their different roles, the actions of the two agents are perceived differently in terms of causal agency and responsibility for death.

By way of further illustration, with more immediate relevance to our present concerns, consider the currently very common view that when physicians withdraw a respirator from a terminal patient who has no hope of recovery, this is a case of permitting death to occur, of allowing natural causes to claim the patient's life. Contrast this with a similar situation in which a well-meaning friend or relative enters the hospital at night and disconnects the respirator. However much one may be inclined to sympathize, excuse, or justify this action, it is much more difficult to insist that it is really only a cause of letting die rather than killing. Similarly, many believe that when physicians order sedation and "nothing by mouth" for a grossly deformed and hopelessly brain-damaged newborn, or when, for similar reasons, they forego the use of antibiotics which would prolong the infant's life, they do not kill it but rather permit it to die, or at most arrange for its death. Yet, surely, most people would think that if a parent were to take a baby like this home, sedate it, and intentionally starve it to death, he or she would have killed it. Moreover, legally, this parent would be liable to charges of homicide through deliberate criminal neglect.

Admittedly, some considerable conceptual and linguistic variation persists in relation to cases of these kinds. Nevertheless, to the extent that these and similar examples represent increasingly prevalent practice, they testify to the way normative considerations, associated with roles and relations, sometimes operate decisively in the very application of the killing/letting die distinction. More specifically, our judgments and determinations of causal agency in death often reflect specifically moral presumptions and standards concerning how a person in a given role *should* have acted.[3]

Returning to the standard argument about moral relevance, what is to show that the sheer difference between killing and letting die never itself makes a moral difference? It is supposed to be the fact that when cases are compared in which intentions, motives, and outcomes all remain constant, and the only difference concerns the causal means of death, one can discover no moral difference between those acts considered in themselves. This clearly presupposes that we can always differentiate killing form letting die in a way that does not itself reflect moral norms. Yet the crucial matter of causal agency, which divides killing from letting die, is often quite sensitive to socially shared role norms and standards having a definite moral force. Therefore, the standard argument of irrelevance becomes untenable by assuming that the killing/letting die distinction is itself morally neutral, when in fact it is not.

While the above may be effective against the letter of the standard argument against the moral relevance of the killing/letting die distinction, it may be thought unfair to its intent and spirit. To assess the position fairly, one will have to hold matters of social role and relation constant, as well as the factors of motive, intention, and outcome. Thus, the central claim will now be that when social and professional roles and relations are the same, and intentions, motives, and outcomes are the same, there can be no moral difference between instances of killing and letting die. Even though the form and degree of causal involvement in the death are different, this bare difference in causal agency cannot, in and of itself, make any relevant difference in moral quality and evaluation.

Conclusions on relevance. My own inclination is to think that the central claim in question betrays a seriously truncated notion of moral *relevance*. Relevance is necessarily relational, and, in general, some factor is relevant to a moral decision or evaluation through its relation to some proposition about consequences, or some principle, rule, or important value. Even deception, or misinformation, or failure to obtain consent in medical contexts, for example, are not just in and of themselves relevant to ethical evaluation. Obviously, these are relevant in relation to certain principles concerning autonomy, self-determination, the dignity of the person, and so forth. With this in mind, it appears that the issue of the moral relevance of the killing/letting die distinction, even under the strictures of the present formulation, simply cannot be decided independently of empirical issues about long-term social consequences. If it is true that allowing some form of active euthanasia, for example, will lead to misapplication and abuse, then there legitimately ought to be moral and legal norms prohibiting this practice. And if there ought to be such prohibitions framing and governing medical practice, then the killing/letting die distinction will be relevant in morally evaluating what physicians do concerning life and death. In short, although it may well be true that moral responsibility and accountability for a *particular* death are equivalent between killing and letting die under the specified conditions, this does not exhaust the possibilities of moral relevance for this distinction. There could still be important social reasons for preferring the one form of responsibility over the other, and this would preserve moral relevance. Consider, for example, a practice which permits killing when some form of passively allowing death would be equally effective in securing desired ends. Responsibility for death may be the same in either case while the passive measures remain morally preferable simply because they minimize exceptions to a rule against homicide.

The first phase of the preceding argument is intended to show that the practical logic of the killing/letting die distinction can importantly depend upon antecedent moral prescriptions governing roles and relations. How could a distinction that may itself turn on moral presuppositions fail to be sometimes relevant to overall moral assessment? The second phase of the argument considers an amended formulation of the standard argument of irrelevance that accommodates the normative force of the distinction itself. However, this formulation only serves to leave us with the central question of what norms and standards ought to frame and govern medical practice regarding causal involvement in death. Ultimately, the entire debate over the moral relevance of the killing/letting die distinction, though interesting and instructive, turns out to be largely trivial. For one cannot argue from any of the common claims concerning moral irrelevance to any conclusions about permissible medical practice, because conclusions about the latter are necessary to determine the truth of the former. And, obviously, these conclusions depend upon complex considerations of the social consequences of allowing the practice of active killing, in terms of general social welfare, human security, and the like. It may or may not be true that some practices involving killing in medical contexts would be legitimate in these terms. There may be completely justifiable medical practices involving such a direct and prominent degree of causal agency in death that they cannot be assimilated in currently recognized instances of allowing death to occur, and therefore must be seen as killing. Nothing in what has been said here rules this out. Rather, my central contention has been that, aside from forcing the rejection of an uncritical assumption that killing *must* involve greater moral responsibility for death than letting die, the current form of debate over the moral relevance of this distinction is itself largely irrelevant to the important issue of what physicians morally should and should not be allowed to do concerning life and death.

COMPARING THE CANADIAN AND U.S. REPORTS

The U.S. Commission report on foregoing life-sustaining treatment and related issues is more comprehensive in treatment and more detailed in argument than its Canadian counterpart. At the level of general principles and conclusions on the particular issues of cessation of treatment and euthanasia, however, there is substantial agreement between them. Both studies forcefully affirm a principle of patient autonomy, giving all competent patients the right to make final decisions about whether to accept available life-sustaining treatment. This principle is constrained in application only by consideration of very serious harm to others or the imposition of unfair burdens on them. In terms of principle, moreover, both reports emphasize that while the presumption concerning incompetent patients should always be that they would want any treatment that would be therapeutically useful for them, the question of usefulness and benefit is not limited to what will merely extend biological existence. Rather, this question must appropriately include consideration of the human meaningfulness and quality of the life that is prolonged.

Ambiguity in the Canadian report. Unfortunately, however, on this crucial point a certain vacillation and ambiguity lurks persistently within the Canadian study, both in its form as a working paper and in the much shorter final report. Let us consider the working paper first. Despite its affirmation that the principle that quality of life considerations must appropriately enter into decisions about the usefulness of treatments, the tendency of all the ensuing explanations and examples is to support an altogether different thesis. They merely illustrate a contrast between treatments offering some hope of improving or at least controlling the course of a disease that untreated would lead to death, and treatments pointlessly prolonging an inevitable process of dying. Summarizing its view of when continued treatment would not serve the patient's overall welfare, the commission says, "In other words, it is not the case when treatment is diverted from its proper end and merely prolongs the dying process rather than life itself" (Working Paper, 59). The problem here is that this seems to leave no real place for the operation of the very fundamental quality of life considerations that are affirmed in principle. For clearly there are cases where the progression of a disease can, in a sense, be controlled, in that death can be staved off for a very long time although there may remain no reasonable hope of regaining any meaningful level of human functioning. For example, there may be no hope of recovering levels of conscious functioning that would permit recognition of, response to, and relationships with others, or any sort of purposive bodily mobility. These kinds of considerations, concerning prospects for physical mobility and purposive behaviour, emotional interrelationships and response, and levels of awareness of self and the world, are what are critical in quality of life judgments. And these sorts of considerations may appropriately declare the therapeutic uselessness of treatment regardless of the fact that some treatment may control or arrest what would otherwise be a condition ending in death. The Canadian Commission Working Paper recognizes no such instances of the application of quality of life judgments. Rather, the overall thrust of its argument is to allow cessation of treatment for incompetents only when treatment uselessly prolongs a dying process. Thus, its principal concern is not so much with quality of life as it is normally understood, but with the quality of an irreversible process of dying. And the effect of its main arguments is really to limit narrowly the scope of what is "therapeutically useless" treatment to what merely prolongs an already inevitable death.[4]

On the other hand, a few statements in the final report seem rather clearly to support the relevance and legitimacy of quality of life judgments in discontinuing treatment for some extreme cases in which continued treatment could sustain biological life. In other words, the final report seems to acknowledge, or at least to suggest, that therapeutically useless treatment may encompass treatment prolonging life at a level of functioning that is unacceptably low. For example, it states: "A decision that would only prolong the dying patient's agony would not be reasonable in the Commission's opinion; nor would a decision be reasonable which would force a newborn or adult to undergo an exceptional series of operations or treatments, resulting in great suffering, only to end up with a medically unacceptable quality of life" (Final Report, 25). This if far from decisive, however, partly because it is unclear what is meant by a "medically unacceptable" quality of life, and partly because these writers conceive themselves to be merely recapitulating what was said in the working paper.

Ultimately, then, there is a notable irony in the Canadian Commission's final recommendation for certain changes in the criminal code making it unambiguously clear that a physician should not incur any criminal liability for discontinuing treatment for an incompetent person when it is no longer therapeutically useful in the person's best interest. Given the discrepancy between their affirmation of the general principle and the preponderant effect of their explanations and examples, it remains quite ambiguous and unclear how we are to understand this recommendation itself, especially concerning the scope of considerations used to determine what is therapeutically useful or useless.

Principle of substituted judgment – U.S. report. By contrast, the U.S. report clearly and consistently upholds a principle of substituted judgment for those unable to decide for themselves. Relying on previous patient testimony and evidence from families and friends, the principle of substituted judgment seeks to determine what the patient would most probably want for himself or herself. Failing this, there is recourse to the consideration of what is in the patient's best interest in a general way. These efforts at determination may centrally involve quality of life considerations concerning forms and levels of both physical and mental functioning (U.S. Commission Report, ch. 4). Regarding procedures for implementing this principle in practice, the report gives a rather prominent and authoritative voice to closely related family members. In contrast, the Canadian report strongly advises consultation with family but gives primary authority to physicians. In accord with these differences, each report sees in very different ways the value and function of so-called living wills and other formal pre-declarations of patient preferences. Both studies naturally emphasize the ultimately determinative role of the courts in unprecedented or unusually problematic cases, and in cases of sharp conflict in opinion between family and physicians.

Rejection of active euthanasia. Finally, and most importantly for our purposes, both reports emphatically recommend against the legal sanction of any forms of active euthanasia, whether voluntary or not, and against any changes in present legal statutes intended to weaken culpability for mercy killing, or having the effect of recognizing compassion as a defence against homicide. Moreover, the reason given for rejecting active euthanasia is essentially the same for both commissions, that is, the risk that weakening present legal prohibitions against deliberately taking life in extreme circumstances would lead to wholly unjustified taking of life in less extreme circumstances. The Canadian report also specifically argues against the decriminalization of any activities aiding or assisting in suicide, although it expresses sympathy for the motives that often prompt these actions.

Remarkably little argument or evidence of any kind is offered by either commission to substantiate the pivotal claim about the risk of abuse, and the erosion of proper respect for human life, which active euthanasia supposedly presents. The Canadian report, to its credit, does briefly compare Anglo-American legal experience and traditions concerning homicide with those of some other countries, such as Switzerland, where compassionate motives are recognized in defence. But the commission finds no grounds for recommending significant change. The deficiency in argument is especially glaring in the U.S. report. For, unlike its counterpart, this commission carefully considers and rejects all the common arguments intended to show some intrinsic moral difference between killing and letting die. In keeping with the foregoing analysis, they appear to accept that when roles and relations are the same, intentions and motives the same or equally acceptable, and outcomes equally certain, moral responsibility for death is completely equal between killing and letting die (U.S. Commission Report, 65–73). Presumably, these writers are acutely aware of how conceptually critical is the empirical claim of risk and long-term social disutility in defending their prohibition of active killing in all medical circumstances. Yet this proposition is simply accepted and pronounced without argument or explanation.

Problem of pointless suffering. Conceivably, of course, practical realism about effecting social change may partially account for this specific indifference to argument. Besides this, however, there are two very important subsidiary aspects of these reports that may help explain and mitigate this deficiency. Both studies recognize that a serious, countervailing consequence of maintaining the legal prohibitions against direct killing of terminally ill patients could be the pointless prolongation of extreme agony and indignity. In response to this problem, both studies strongly emphasize that it is not immoral, and often a positive obligation, strenuously to employ analgesic drugs and procedures for the control of suffering, even when their use may hasten death. The Law Reform Commission, again, recommends changes in the criminal code to remove any ambiguity about this. Thus, both reports rely heavily on the possibility of relieving the harms of agony and suffering through aggressive palliative care rather than through changes in the laws against homicide. An important conceptual point in this connection is that aggressive pain-relieving therapy, even when it dramatically hastens death, can be protected against the charge that it is actually killing through the distinction between directly intended consequences and consequences that are foreseen but unintended. For these cases, the important primary intention is to control suffering, while the hastening of death is an acceptable and foreseeable consequence of it.

In response, it can reasonably be doubted that even the most vigorous analgesic therapy directed at the control of physical pain can adequately relieve all of the most serious forms of suffering, such as continuous breathlessness, nausea, endless vomiting, incontinence, and the rapid decline of mental powers and functions. Obviously, such therapy could certainly deal with these problems if drug dosages were permitted at positively lethal levels. But this would clearly be equivalent to active euthanasia under the guise of pain control, since the crucial distinction between intended and merely foreseen consequences would collapse. For if we can use something intending to control pain, but at a level we foresee will immediately cause death, then we face the unanswerable question of why we cannot use something intending to cause death because we foresee that this will immediately relieve suffering.

Finally, there is a second important reason why the U.S. Commission in particular takes a relatively sanguine attitude about the possibility of meeting all or most legitimate compassionate and humanitarian objectives in medicine without any change in present prohibitions against direct killing. This report specifically includes artificial means of providing foods and fluids within the range of medical technologies that may legitimately be withdrawn when they no longer serve any therapeutic purpose (U.S. Commission Report, 89–90, 132–36, 189–90). Although the Canadian report is silent on this question, nothing that is said rules it out either. In any case, perhaps nothing is more germane today to the issue of whether we genuinely need radical moral and legal reform than the question of whether the withholding of nutrition and hydration can legitimately be included with other recognized and morally acceptable practices of foregoing or withholding medical treatments. For clearly, if this can be regarded as a passive measure, on a par with others, then many patients whose lives might otherwise have to be sustained indefinitely become potential candidates for compassionate non-treatment. I will close with a consideration of this issue.

THE MORALITY OF WITHHOLDING FOOD AND FLUID

Are we ever justified in withholding or withdrawing foods and fluids in terminal or other cases? This issue has two main aspects. First, can the provision of nutrition be regarded as medical treatment to be evaluated on a par with other treatment modalities, such as artificial respiration or dialysis? Or is the provision of food always a matter of basic nursing care, the value of which must be seen in expressive and symbolic terms extending beyond specific benefit to an individual patient? Second, and more fundamentally, if homicide is essentially the intentional causing of death, how are we to avoid this classification for the intentional withdrawing of nutrition leading to death? In short, is recognizing the legitimacy of sometimes withdrawing food and fluid tantamount to sanctioning killing in medical settings? This paper argues that the provision of nutrition in the relevant cases is properly evaluated as medical treatment and that the classification as killing can properly be avoided.

The issue of symbolic value. The basic standard governing treatment decisions for incompetent patients, upheld by both the U.S. President's Commission and the Canadian Law Reform Commission in their studies on foregoing treatment, is one requiring the general advancement of the patient's interests when patient preferences cannot be known (U.S. Commission Report, ch. 4; Canadian Working Paper, part 3, sec. 3). It is by now very generally accepted in medical practice that this principle can sometimes justify the termination of medical treatment, when such treatment does not serve the patient's welfare. But if this principle can sometimes justify non-resuscitation, withholding dialysis or transfusions, withdrawing a respirator, and so forth, then it is certainly natural to think that it could likewise justify instances of withholding or withdrawing intravenous or nasogastric nutrition. Accordingly, a strong current of moral thought has developed recently which holds that artificial means of providing food and water are inherently no different from other medical treatments and that their use should be evaluated by this same principle. Cases are pointed to in which artificial nutrition and hydration are as useless to patient welfare as other medical technologies for whose withdrawal a moral consensus already exists. Thus, in the case of a patient in a permanent vegetative state, as was Karen Quinlan, or in the case of an anencephalic infant, it could be argued that the same reasons concerning patient welfare that would justify withholding a respirator would also justify withholding feeding and hydration tubes. Or consider an infant with virtually no bowel formation. Gastrointestinal methods are mostly futile because so little nutrient is absorbed, and intravenous methods will probably lead eventually, in weeks or months to complications like thrombosis and infection, causing death.

An opposing tendency of moral thought holds that we are always obliged to provide nutrition and hydration, even in hopeless cases, because these activities symbolize or express the essence of care and compassion. Such actions should not be assessed simply in the light of goals and objectives in an individual case, but should also be seen in terms of what they symbolically communicate concerning basic human and professional values. A powerful medical tradition insists upon the duty to give basic nursing care and comfort to patients, even when nothing of therapeutic value can be done for them. Allowing the withdrawal of food and fluid, under any circumstances, would weaken the force of this tradition of providing basic care even when nothing more can be done. And this could have unfortunate effects on the most fundamental terms of the relationship between the medical profession and patients.

In the remainder of this section I will try to develop a middle course between these extremes, that is, between the belief that artificially supplied food and water can never be withdrawn morally and the belief that, other things being equal, they can be withdrawn anytime we are justified in foregoing other life-sustaining treatments.

Against the claim for special symbolic and expressive value in always providing food and fluid one can range an equally powerful prevalent and opposite perception. Specifically technological means of supplying nutrition and hydration do not always successfully convey the essence of care and compassion. Unlike the image of a cool hand upon a fevered brow, or of a patient being delicately spoon-fed, the sight of nasogastric tubes in therapeutically futile situations often produces an exactly contrary suggestive effect. In these circumstances, such efforts suggest to many who have witnessed them a kind of rigid adherence to institutional routines and policies regardless of their therapeutic pointlessness, and sometimes even regardless of the pain and indignity they prolong for the individual. Imagine, for example, an elderly patient in the terminal stages of an extremely debilitating and painful cancer, whose relatives' compassionate requests that he not be sustained by artificial feeding are ignored in the interests of unalterable policy or principle.

The point here is that it does no logical good simply to insist that always supplying nutrition upholds an important symbolic value when the actual experience of many people in witnessing these activities, in certain extreme circumstances, undermines this claim. Whose reactions or moral intuitions are we to trust? Besides, does this whole issue reduce merely to an impasse between contrary forms of moral sensibility or perception, some seeing symbolic value maintained where others see pointless moral conservatism?

Perhaps more progress can be made by qualifying the "par-value" position in a way that preserves something of the intent and spirit of the "symbolic-value" position. The first view has two parts that are usually, but unnecessarily, run together. First it claims that artificial provision of food and water is on a moral par with other medical treatments and should be evaluated in the same terms, and then it concludes that such provision of food and water morally can be foregone just as, and whenever, other life-sustaining treatments can be stopped. Understandably, this conclusion troubles many people. For one may be prepared to countenance non-feeding in certain extreme cases – such as a terminal case in which artificial feeding prolongs a very burdensome process of dying, or in the case of an irreversibly comatose patient for whom continued biological life can have no value – but not accept it as a potential moral option just because *some* life-sustaining treatment morally could be foregone. Consider a case of irreversible, progressive dementia in an aged person who is not terminal. Suppose her condition renders her dysfunctional and debilitated, though not utterly vegetative, and places her beyond the reach of all but the most rudimentary communications. Interpersonal relations are impossible and perhaps it is even doubtful whether any sense of personal identity survives at all. On the view we are considering, one could not consistently hold, for this case, that it would be morally legitimate to forego, say, antibiotic therapy in the face of life-threatening sepsis, or chemotherapy for some controllable cancer, while at the same time morally rejecting discontinuation of artificial feeding. Yet it would be very helpful in the current debate over withdrawing food and water if the logical opportunity for this kind of compromise position were recognized clearly.

We must note first that from the claim that artificial feeding is on a par with other medical treatments and should be morally evaluated in the same terms, it does not necessarily follow that non-feeding must be all right, other things being equal, whenever it would be all right to forego other life-preserving treatments. Whether this follows or not depends upon exactly what the operative terms of evaluation are to be. Naturally, the principal focus has been on individual patient interest and welfare. But we are asking about a matter of general medical practice or policy, namely, under what conditions can artificial feeding morally be stopped? As the "symbolic-value" view recognizes in its own way, we cannot properly consider this issue without taking the social consequences of general policy into account. Our terms of evaluation therefore include both patient welfare and social consequences. For this reason, it may be true that artificial feeding should be evaluated in the *same terms* as other life-sustaining technologies, while it is false that nutrition can therefore morally be withdrawn under all the same conditions as the latter, other things being equal in the particular case. Significant differences in expectable social consequences at the level of general policy must be part of this comparative evaluation.

We know that two definable groups of patients have disproportionately high representation among those requiring artificial nutrition and hydration, namely seriously compromised or defective newborns and the very debilitated and fragile old. Some patients in these groups certainly could be beneficiaries of a general policy permitting the withdrawal of food and water in certain circumstances. But, at the same time, we have to recognize that these patient groups are especially vulnerable to mistreatment and abuse. They are generally powerless while being frequently burdensome and expensive. Since anyone will die without food and water, providing appropriate protection for these groups arguably entails extreme caution and rigour in the formulation of general, morally justifying conditions and procedures for the removal of artificial nutrition. In this way, one could consistently recognize the moral legitimacy of foregoing other life-sustaining technologies in various circumstances, while insisting that the general conditions justifying the withdrawal of food and fluid have to be maximally stringent and limited. For non-voluntary cases, perhaps these limits should extend only to terminal cases in which continued life would be very painful and burdensome, or cases involving merely vegetative existence without prospects for consciousness.

On this view, then, it is not that artificially supplying nutrition has a symbolic value that must be upheld at all costs. Nor is it that there is simply no moral basis for a distinction between artificial feeding and other technological means of sustaining life. The conjunction of the universal necessity of food and water for continued life and the special vulnerability of certain patient groups, particularly defective newborns and the very fragile old, provides the ground for especially stringent moral conditions for withdrawing nutrition and hydration.[5]

The issue of homicide. Our second question concerning artificial nutrition and hydration is whether their removal can logically avoid classification as homicide. Presumably, if this cannot be done, current legal and medical prohibitions of active killing in any form will serve to condemn such a practice, whatever might be said in its favour.

Partially reflecting the view of the immediately preceding section, several U.S. courts have ruled that the removal of intravenous or gastrointestinal tubes is not essentially different from the removal of other medical modalities, and that their benefits and burdens ought to be evaluated in the same way. (We have seen here that it is not the terms of evaluation that are said to make a moral difference between removing nutrition tubes and stopping other forms of life-sustaining treatment. Rather, it is the differential results of the application of one of those terms, namely, consideration of social consequences.) This judgment is well illustrated by the 1983 California case of *Barber and Nejdle* v. *Superior Court 2*. Acting on the request of the family, Drs. Barber and Nejdle first removed a respirator and then intravenous tubes from Clarence Herbert, who had suffered severe brain damage after a cardiac arrest. As the result of a dispute with someone on the support staff, criminal charges were laid against them. The court ruled that their action, under the circumstantances, was not an affirmative act constituting unlawful killing but rather an omission justified by Mr. Herbert's condition and prospects. Moreover, the court argued specifically that medical procedures to provide nutrition and hydration are completely on a par with other medical procedures and are to be evaluated in the same manner.[6]

In a comparable case, however, a New Jersey appeals court recently found the opposite on the question of homicide. Mrs. Conroy, aged eighty-three, suffered from severe organic brain syndrome and advanced diabetes. She was virtually unable to move, she could not communicate and had lost all capacity for cognitive and rational functioning. Consequent to the diabetes, she developed necrotic ulcers on her left foot and it was recommended that her left leg be amputated. Her guardian refused permission for the operation and also petitioned the court to have her nasogastric tube removed. This petition was granted but the decision was stayed pending appeal. Shortly thereafter, Mrs. Conroy died with the tube still in place. In July 1983, an appeals court reversed the lower court's decision. Despite Mrs. Conroy's condition and prospects, this court did not view the case as one of forgoing medical treatment, but as one in which Mrs. Conroy would have been purposefully killed by being starved. "If the trial judge's order had been enforced, Conroy would not have died as the result of an existing medical condition, but rather she would have died, and painfully so, as the result of a new and independent condition: dehydration and starvation. Thus she would have been killed by independent means."[7]

Before confronting the homicide issue, it is important to note that if pain and suffering would result from removing nutrition and hydration tubes in a case in which it would otherwise be justified, this difficulty could normally be met by aggressive analgesic therapy. This approach would be consistent, as we have seen, with both the Law Reform Commission and the Presidential Commission reports, which insist on the legitimacy of sedation, even at levels which hasten death, if this is necessary to control suffering after a decision to forego some life-sustaining treatment.

Comparison with Quinlan. Thus the critical issue that emerges is whether the withdrawal of nutrition and hydration, in cases of the type under consideration, must be seen as homicide, as held by the New Jersey appellate court. It will be helpful to consider this question in relation to the extreme case of the pre-terminal, permanently comatose patient. The *Quinlan* decision holds that the removal of a respirator from a permanently comatose patient is not the primary and significant cause of death; the death is to be seen as the result of pre-existing natural causes. Yet removing a respirator and depriving a patient of oxygen certainly are material causal conditions of death. Nevertheless, the logic of this watershed legal decision has largely prevailed, yielding the currently common view that when physicians withdraw a respirator from a terminal patient or from a patient existing without any prospect of recovering humanly meaningful life, this is a case of permitting death to occur, of allowing natural causes to claim the patient's life.

We are thus brought back to the matter we discussed at the beginning, the way and extent to which this common mode of thinking forces us to recognize that normative and moral standards concerning what physicians may or should do are operating decisively in the determination of causal role and agency in death, upon which the classification of homicide depends. For consider again how the situation would be viewed if a friend or relative took it upon themselves surreptitiously to disconnect the respirator from a patient in a hopeless condition. Legally speaking, this emphatically would not be regarded as a merely passive action, as merely allowing the patient to die of pre-existing causes, as in the *Quinlan* case. As we found before, our judgments and determinations of causal agency in death, which are at the heart of the question of homicide, often reflect specific moral presumptions and standards concerning how a person in a given role should have acted.

This way of reasoning, which avoids classifying physicians' withholding or withdrawing of certain life-sustaining treatments as homicide, is related to the legal doctrine of "proximate" cause. Though analyses of this concept are various and complex, one prominent interpretation holds that for an agent to be the "proximate" or principal cause of an outcome is for the agent to do something upon which legal responsibility for the outcome can be founded. The issue of responsibility in turn depends upon the agent's duties and obligations. In the case, therefore, where there is no obligation to initiate or continue treatment, the tendency of the law will be to locate the principal cause of death in the course of pathological events leading to death, even though this sequence may be conditioned by non-treatment.

In light of this, what is the most reasonable answer to the question of whether withdrawing artificial feeding can properly avoid classification as homicide? It would appear that the very same logic that protects the removal of a respirator from this classification can be applied, point for point, in the instance of withdrawing artificial nutrition and hydration. Consider the strictness of the analogy between these actions in the case of the permanently comatose patient. Both procedures may constitute a material causal condition of death; and both may involve the same intention and the same degree of moral responsibility. If removing the respirator avoids classification as homicide because the existing pathology is seen as the primary of "proximate" cause of death, why should we not view removing a nasogastric tube in the same way? In either case, without continued intervention, the patient's disease can be said to claim the life, through a fatal oxygen deficit in the one case, and through a fatal nutritional and hydrational deficit in the other. And the critically important thing in both cases is that neither procedure can cure, or improve, or ameliorate the patient's fundamental condition, which may be seen as cancelling any duty to provide them.

While the presumption in medicine must always be that incompetent patients would want any treatment that would be therapeutically useful for them, the question of usefulness and benefit is not limited nowadays to what will merely extend biological existence. Socially and legally we have come to accept that therapeutic pointlessness, in terms of the *quality* of life that is prolonged, sometimes cancels any obligation to continue respiration. Given the prevailing logic of the *Quinlan* decision, if we should decide socially that it is *desirable* for physicians to forgo artificial nutrition in some cases, then the formula is already at hand for classifying this also as a passive procedure.

Ultimately, the question of the morality of withholding artificial nutrition and hydration depends upon what policy will most benefit us. We must directly confront this fundamental issue of what *is* desirable, individually and socially, without illusions regarding the power of either medical traditions of providing ordinary care and comfort, or legal prohibitions of active killing, to short-circuit this inquiry.

NOTES

1 This paper includes revised material from two earlier papers of mine, "Decisions about Life and Death," *Journal of Medical Humanities and Bioethics,* vol. 6, no. 2, 1985, and "The Morality of Withholding Food and Fluid," *Journal of Palliative Care,* vol. 3, no. 2, 1987.

2 The classic statement and elaboration of this argument against the moral relevance of the killing/letting die distinction per se is James Rachels, "Active and Passive Euthanasia," *New England Journal of Medicine,* vol. 78, 1975.

3 For the classic analysis of judgments of causation in practical life see H. L. A. Hart and A. M. Honore, *Causation in the Law,* Oxford: Oxford University Press 1959. Hart and Honore recognize various ways in which practical judgments of causation are conditioned by normative standards and presuppositions. But see especially 35ff.

4 These points are best appreciated by consulting the statement of general principles contained in the Working Paper, part 3, particularly section 3, and the discussion of cases in part 4, section 3.

5 Writing in a very different vein, Daniel Callahan has recently suggested a similar compromise concerning the specific issue of feeding the dying elderly. See his "Feeding the Dying Elderly," *Generations,* Winter 1985, 16.

6 *Barber and Nejdle* v. *Sup. Ct. 2,* Civil No. 69350, 69351, Ct. of App. 2nd Dist., Div. 2, 12 October 1983. This case is reviewed in considerable detail in Bonnie Steinbock, "The Removal of Mr. Herbert's Feeding Tube," *Hastings Center Report,* vol. 13, no. 5, October 1983.

7 "In the Matter of Conroy," Sup. Ct. NJ App. Div., A2483-82, 8 July 1983. I take this quotation from George Annas, "Nonfeeding: Lawful Killing in CA, Homicide in NJ," *Hastings Center Report,* vol. 13, no. 6, December 1983. Annas contrasts and comments upon *Barber and Nejdle* and *Conroy,* but without reaching any firm conclu-

sions. The case of Conroy has since been reviewed by the New Jersey Supreme Court, which, with extensive qualification, has upheld the original ruling.

REFERENCES

Law Reform Commission of Canada. *Euthanasia, Aiding Suicide and Cessation of Treatment*. Working Paper 28. Ottawa: Minister of Supply and Services 1982. Also, the Commission's final report, no. 20, of the same title (1983)

President's Commission for the Study of Ethical Problems in Medicine and Biomedical and Behavioral Research. *Deciding to Forego Life-sustaining Treatment: Ethical, Medical and Legal Issues in Treatment Decisions*. Washington, DC: U.S. Government Printing Office 1983

12

Foregoing Life-Sustaining Treatment: The Canadian Law Reform Commission and the President's Commission

ALISTER BROWNE

Modern medicine has dramatically raised our quality of life and our life expectancy. It has also raised some vexing moral problems. In the past, there was seldom any question of doctors *deciding* to let patients die, for it was generally not within their power to keep them alive. Today this situation is changed; thanks to new and improved knowledge, technology, drugs, and surgical techniques, doctors often have the ability to keep patients alive, seemingly indefinitely. The problem is that this is not always a benefit to the patient, and hence doctors have a moral problem they did not have before: since death is avoidable, its occurrence must be the result of a moral decision. Thus the questions arise: "Under what conditions, if any, can treatment necessary for life be withheld or withdrawn?" and "Who is to make that decision?" These questions were addressed by the Canadian Law Reform Commission (CLRC) in its Working Paper, *Euthanasia, Aiding Suicide and Cessation of Treatment,*[1] and Final Report of the same title,[2] and by the United States' President's Commission for the Study of Ethical Problems in Medicine and Biomedical and Behavioral Research (PC) in its report, *Deciding to Forego Life-sustaining Treatment.*[3] In what follows, I will compare and critically evaluate their answers.

CURRENT LEGAL SITUATION

The law in both Canada and the United States agree that one who is competent can refuse any treatment, whatever the consequences, and any attempt to force it upon that person constitutes assault. In the United States, a number of court decisions, including perhaps most famously *Quinlan*[4] and *Saikewicz,*[5] have made it clear that if the patient is incompetent, maximally aggressive treatment need not be continued to the end. The exact conditions under which treatment can be foregone have not been settled once and for all, but the law is firm and clear on the point that life-preserving treatment may be omitted when that is a reasonable course of action.

By contrast, Canadian law is ambiguous in the case of the incompetent patient. Taken literally, section 197 of the Criminal Code tells us that no treatment necessary for life can be withheld, and section 199 that no treatment necessary for life can be withdrawn. Thus, if we take these sections at face value, it appears we must give maximally aggressive treatment until a patient is dead, and some legal experts read the law in just this way. The Canadian Law Reform Commission, however, takes a different view. It contends that sections 197 and 199 should not be read in isolation, but rather in conjunction with the negligence provisions of the Code, and, thus read, the law allows for withholding or withdrawing treatment if that is reasonable; other legal experts interpret the law in this way.

Mr. Justice Lloyd G. McKenzie had an opportunity to offer a resolution of this indeterminacy in the Supreme Court of B.C. decision in *Dawson,*[6] a case over whether surgery must be performed, contrary to the family's wishes, to repair a life-support shunt on a seven-year-old boy with serious neurological problems and a poor prognosis. But he did not dare to be clear. At one point he interpreted the law in a conservative way, when he excluded as legally irrelevant quality of life considerations, writing that: "I do not think that it lies within the prerogative of any parent or of the court to look down upon a disadvantaged person and judge the quality of that person's life to be so low as not to be deserving of continuance" (184). But at another point, he argued that treatment in the case of Stephen Dawson must be continued because the life projected for the child did not plainly fall below an acceptable level, thus implying that life is not always sacred, and that quality of life considerations are relevant. After commenting, "I am satisfied that the laws of our society are structured to preserve, protect and maintain human life and that in the exercise of its inherent jurisdiction this court could not sanction the termination of a life except for the most coercive reasons . . . " (183), Mr. Justice McKenzie went on to argue that there were no such reasons present in the case of Stephen Dawson:

> To refer back to the words of Templeman, L.J. I cannot in conscience find that this is a case of severe proved damage "where the future is so uncertain and where the life of the child is so bound to be full of pain and suffering that the court might be driven to a different conclusion." I am not satisfied that "the life of this child is demonstrably going to be so awful that in effect the

> child must be condemned to die." Rather, I believe that "the life of this child is so imponderable that it would be wrong for her to be condemned to die. (187)

It is in this unsatisfactorily uncertain state that Canadian law currently rests.

RECOMMENDATIONS ON FOREGOING TREATMENT

Both commissions clearly and forcefully endorse the principle of self-determination, according to which if persons are unencumbered, then, insofar as they do not harm or threaten harm to others, they can lay out their own existences as they see fit. This underwrites their recommendations that there be no change in the law with respect to the competent individual's right to refuse treatment. The CLRC does, however, recommend reform in the case of withholding/withdrawing treatment from the incompetent, urging that it clearly be acknowledged that this can sometimes be done without criminal liability. But it dithers on the question of when treatment can be foregone.

In its Working Paper, the CLRC first addresses in a robustly liberal way the question of when treatment can be withheld/withdrawn, contending that the law "must admit that the cessation or noninitiation of treatment which offers no chance of success is *a good decision and one based on sound medical practice*" (italics theirs, 58). It goes on to add that "the guiding principle for medical decision-making is not life itself as an absolute value, but the patient's overall welfare" (59), and proceeds to specify instances in which it is not the case that the patient's overall welfare dictates maintaining life: "It is not the case when the prolonging of life has become purely artificial. It is not the case when the maintenance of life can only be achieved by an undue prolongation of the patient's agony. It is not the case when the maintenance of life results only in the infliction of additional suffering" (59).

But having said this, the Commission immediately muddies the waters by writing: "In other words, it is not the case when treatment is diverted from its proper end and merely prolongs the dying process rather than life itself" (59). The problem is that this is manifestly not a paraphrase of what precedes, for the preceding does not exclusively refer to dying patients whereas the paraphrase does, and thus a conservative element is introduced which suggests that treatment can be foregone only in the case of the dying. This conservatism is reinforced on the next page when the Commission rejects the legitimacy of withholding necessary surgery from a child suffering from Down's syndrome because that involves making "a value judgment as to the quality of the infant's present or future life" (60), and thus seems to exclude, as illegitimate, withholding treatment for quality of life reasons when treatment will preserve life.

In its Final Report, however, the CLRC returns to its liberal stand. It unabashedly speaks of the appropriateness of withholding/withdrawing treatment which does not offer reasonable hope for an "acceptable quality of life," and recommends "that a physician should not incur any criminal liability if he decides to discontinue or not initiate treatment for an incompetent person, when that treatment is no longer therapeutically useful and is not in the person's best interest" (27–28). But how we are to understand this is far from clear, partly because the writers of the Final Report take themselves to be merely recapitulating what was said in the Working Paper, and partly because the examples they offer in the Final Report only partially support a liberal reading. After having offered the recommendation quoted above, the CLRC goes on:

> This would be the case [i.e., that treatment is not therapeutically useful and not in the patient's best interest], for example, when artificial ventilation was continued for a patient whose cerebral functions had already undergone irreversible cessation. This would also be the case when a physician, who, in order to avoid prolonging the death agony of one of his patients, decides to discontinue antibiotics being given to treat his pneumonia. A further example would be the case of a surgeon who decides not to operate to correct a newborn's deformity because, even if the operation were successful, the infant could not survive his other medical problems. (34)

The first example certainly liberalizes the "we can only terminate treatment on the dying" motif of the Working Paper, for those who have suffered permanent loss of higher-brain function need not be dying. However, the other examples deal with dying patients, and we are thus still left in the dark as to how the CLRC views foregoing treatment on patients who are not irreversibly comatose, can be treated in a way so as to ensure the continuance of life, but whose lives are of an extremely low quality. There is, then, a certain irony in the CLRC's attempt to clarify the law. Given the ambiguous theory and unhelpful examples, it remains quite unclear as to how we are to understand their recommendations.

By contrast, the President's Commission clearly and consistently upholds a principle of substituted judgment for those unable to decide for themselves, i.e., that, wherever possible, the surrogate attempt to reach the decision that the incapacitated person would make if he or she were able to choose (132), and, where it is not, that the judgment be made on the basis of the patient's best interest, i.e., by reference to more objective societally shared criteria, where this includes factors such as the relief of suffering, the preservation or restoration of functioning, and the quality as well as the extent of life sustained (135). In recommending this, the PC adopts a liberal view on foregoing treatment. By making substituted judgment the controlling concern, it goes beyond limiting foregoing treatment to the dying, for there is a whole range of cases in which a person is not dying but where we have excellent reason to think he would not want to be kept alive. And where substituted judgments are not possible, the criteria it provides for the evaluation of "best interest" judgments allow for the withholding/withdrawing of treatment in cases other than those of the dying.

My view is that the PC is substantially correct. Respect for the autonomy of the individual bids us accept the principle of self-determination according to which competent adults should be free to lay out their existence as they see fit. It does not immediately follow that we must unswervingly accept the principle of substituted judgment once individuals become incompetent. For what persons want may be quite irrational and contrary to their interests, and while there is nothing morally wrong with competent individuals harming themselves for a bad reason, there is something morally wrong with standing by and allowing or assisting incompetent ones to do so. Still, the principle of substituted judgment has force, for respect for autonomy dictates that we cannot shuffle aside the fixed and settled desires which persons have exhibited throughout their competent lives without very weighty reasons. Thus a consistent and rigorous application of the principle of self-determination leads us to a liberal view of termination of treatment, as the PC recommends.

DETERMINING SUBSTITUTED JUDGMENT: LIVING WILLS

In recent years, the idea of living wills – or, as they are technically called in the United States, "Natural Death Acts" – has become popular, and anyone who endorses the priority of substituted judgment must look favourably on them, for they function to project one's desires into a future in which one cannot speak for oneself. The PC accepts this implication, and recommends that living wills receive legal status. But the CLRC is ambivalent. In part 4 of its Working Paper it too recommends that living wills have binding legal force, contending that when patients have expressed their wishes in writing they "should be respected and the doctor is required to adopt the same position as if his patient were conscious and competent" (61). In part 5, however, the CLRC reverses itself, rejecting the concept of a living will, and makes no mention of that form of advance declaration in its Final Report.

This ambivalence can be explained partly by the conservative streak in the CLRC which inclines it to make termination of treatment decisions medical decisions, and partly – and officially – by a curious mischaracterization of living wills. In part 4, the CLRC characterizes them as providing a sufficient condition for terminating treatment, but in part 5 it characterizes them as providing a necessary condition.

> We believe that it would risk the reversal of the already-established rule that there should be no duty to initiate or maintain treatment when it is useless to do so. The living will approach begins from the opposite principle, since it requires that the patient's wishes be formally expressed in writing in order to authorize the physician not to prolong the patient's agony and death. This approach may be arguable in the context and legal systems of California and other States, but we do not feel it is an arguable reform for Canada. (69)

We may well agree that living wills, construed as *necessary* conditions for the termination of useless treatment, would be undesirable, but this does nothing to show the inutility or undesirability of living wills construed as *sufficient* conditions for the termination of certain treatments which would otherwise be continued. But even setting aside the CLRC's official argument as a classic case of a straw man, one may have some doubts about the advisability of living wills.

First, physicians may come to hold the view that if a patient has not made out a living will that is to be construed as a wish for maximally aggressive treatment until the end. Indeed, in California, this seems to have been the effect of their Natural Death Act. The PC reports that while 6.5 per cent of physicians interviewed claimed they omitted treatment they otherwise would have administered, 10 per cent admitted they administered treatment they otherwise would have omitted (144).

Second, it is difficult to give content to the wills in a way that does not make them unnecessary or problematical. If they only specify that useless treatment may be withdrawn from dying patients, they do not go beyond existing law and medical practice, and thus are at best otiose, and at worst dangerous in that they may encourage the aggressive medicine alluded to above. On the other hand, if living wills do go beyond the occasions on which a physician unarmed with any advance declaration would routinely terminate treatment, we are faced with the question of whether they are suitably informed to be legally binding. *Now,* our judgment may be that we do not want to be resuscitated if we are senile and have stopped breathing; *then,* though we may not be able to say so, we may take a different view. And this may put doctors in an awkward situation: a senile patient stops breathing; his living will, made when fully competent and never rescinded, instructs that he does not want to be resuscitated in that event; he nonetheless has exhibited every behavioural indication of rather enjoying life. What is the physician to do? In a straightforward sense, the presence of the living will makes the physician's decision more difficult than it otherwise would have been, and may work contrary to the best interest of the patient.

The PC frankly acknowledges these difficulties, and yet contends, rightly I think, that living wills should be given legal effect. The overtreatment problem can be substantially met by both a clear declaration to the effect that living wills are not necessary conditions for the foregoing of treatment and suitable hospital directives. It is surely not beyond the wit of legislators and hospital directors to write such directives, and doctors to understand them. But even if physicians will sometimes overtreat, that should not be taken as decisive against natural death acts, though it certainly runs counter to their aim. We should not take away the means of self-determination from those who wish to use it just because there are others who will not, and who will be worse off as a result. It should also be noted that overtreatment, especially if supplemented by the kinds of palliative care that both Commissions promise can be and typically is delivered, is, while a fate worse than death, not much so.

There are two replies to the underinformed objection. First, there is the tough line that whenever one is given the right to make a choice one can make a mistake, and if the choice is important, the mistake can be serious. Tragedies sometimes will occur from acting strictly on living wills, but the importance of giving people the decision is so great, and the results generally so good, that that is a price which must be paid. Alternatively, there is the milder line that physicians should have some latitude to set aside the living will in the presence of compelling evidence that the patient would no longer choose that option.

Both lines overcome the objection, but my sympathies lie with the second. There is a straightforward sense in which the incompetent person at T_2 is a different person from the competent one who made the living will at T_1. We can, to be sure, trace the body of the person at T_2 back to the body of the person at T_1, but they are no more the same person than the vicious young psychopath and the gentle and kindly Birdman of Alcatraz were the same person. Why should we let the desires of the former person control the destiny of the latter?

One response is that we should do so because the person at T_1 is competent whereas the one at T_2 is not. But we can give priority to the competent person only if the incompetent one's choice is irrational. If the choices are equally rational, and if the competent person no longer exists, there is no reason whatsoever to do so, and every reason not to. And surely there is nothing irrational about wanting to live when senile when life continues to hold pleasure.

It would, indeed, be odd not to adjust living wills in this way. Proponents of living wills urge their authors to update them each year, and it would be absurd for doctors to hold them to their earlier word. Why should not behavioural evidence of enjoyment be read as countermanding earlier instructions as much as an actual change in the wording of the will? Nor could one rightly object that to allow physicians to override living wills would make them pointless, for the patient's wishes are to be considered binding in the absence of clear behavioural evidence to the contrary.

But there is a question about which I am much less confident: Should penalties for non-compliance be attached to living wills? To have them may well cause a doctor to practise defensive medicine and think more about the law than his patient's interests; and, given the necessarily underinformed nature of advance declarations, this may run counter to both a patient's overall welfare and what he would want, given his new set of desires and expectations. On the other hand, not to attach sanctions puts a person's fixed and settled desires in jeopardy. If relatives oppose a patient's views about termination of treatment, it would be a rare doctor who would risk being taken to court by acting on the living will. Living wills would thus be reduced to instructional declarations with only weak guarantees for the author. With important utilities so evenly divided, a rational decision is impossible. In the United States, ten of the states having natural death acts do not specify penalties, five make the physician liable to a charge of unprofessional conduct.[7] We can only watch with interest this experimental legislation and decide in the light of the outcomes. But whether sanctions are attached or not, recognizing living wills as having the legal force of justifying termination of treatment in certain situations would be a useful safeguard of the autonomy of the individual.

WHO DECIDES FOR THE INCOMPETENT?

There is no way to formalize a set of criteria which will make decisions to forego treatment mechanical. If the patient has made a living will, someone has to decide whether it is to be overridden; if a patient has not, someone has to try to determine, on the basis of substituted judgment if possible, best interest judgment if not, what to do on the patient's behalf. Who has the right, and the awesome responsibility, to make such decisions?

The PC recommends that the decision generally be made jointly by a family member (the PC uses the term "family" in a broad way to cover not only next of kin but also friends and other relatives) and the physician and other health professions. It rejects the idea of mandatory judicial review, as well as that by any more informal body such as a hospital ethics committee. The courts have only the role of adjudicating conflicts between the above (or between the above and some other interested) parties, and the function of ethics committees is limited to providing support and further consultation. Finally, the PC recommends that all parties involved in the decision – from physicians to family to review committees – bear legal responsibility for it.

I am in agreement with all of this. Clearly, we cannot leave the decision to the family alone, for there is a medical component in the decision. Equally clearly, we cannot leave the decision up to the physician for there is a non-medical component in the decision. Indeed, once the medical facts have been duly recognized and appreciated, the family should have the dominant say. The rationale for this, as before, stems from the principle of self-determination. That principle entails that when individuals cannot make their own decisions, others should generally make them on the basis of substituted judgment; this, in turn, entails that those who know the individuals best should make the decisions, and those are typically the family. This, coupled with the facts that the family will generally be most concerned with the welfare of the patient and will have to bear brunt of the decision, strongly suggests that the family generally should have the dominant say. To this basic case, the PC adds three buttressing considerations:

> (1) The family deserves recognition as an important social unit that ought to be treated, within limits, as a responsible decision-maker in matters that intimately affect its members.
> (2) Especially in a society in which many other traditional forms of community have eroded, participation in family is often an important dimension of personal fulfillment.
> (3) Since a protected sphere of privacy and autonomy is required for the flourishing of this interpersonal union, institutions and the state should be reluctant to intrude, particularly regarding matters that are personal and on which there is a wide range of opinion in society. (128)

This case for vesting the decision-making power in the joint hands of family and physician, however, is not decisive. There is still plenty of scope for bad judgment and conflict of interest, and thus one may suggest that there should be a mandatory review procedure. Mandatory judicial review is one option. It was endorsed by the Supreme Court of Massachusetts in *Saikewicz*, and has other supporters.[8] It was, however, opposed by the New Jersey Supreme Court in *Quinlan*,[9] and seems on the whole a bad idea. Courts are already clogged, judges have no special competence to decide questions of foregoing treatment, and an adversarial stance is unsuited to making the best decisions and may cause serious and unfortunate rifts between the family and medical personnel.

There is more to be said for mandatory review by some less formal body, such as an ethics committee, but here too there is a down side. For one thing, we increase bureaucracy with all its attendant evils. The joking definition of a camel is a horse designed by committee, and it is not clear that death by committee will have any more pleasing a shape. Nor is it clear that we will get any better decisions; indeed, there is some reason to fear the reverse. There is a danger that ethics committees will degenerate into debating forums. There is also a fear that political aims may intrude, and this is exacerbated if special-interest advocates are given a place on the committee: emphasis may shift from what would be in *this* patient's interest to what would be in the interest of a *class* of patients, and this may work to a particular patient's detriment. Diffusing responsibility may result in no one's feeling personally responsible for the decision, and thus it may not be taken as seriously as it should. Finally, diluting the judgment of the family takes matters out of the hands of those most knowledgeable and concerned about the patient and who will typically have to bear the brunt of the decision, and this is likely to compromise the quality of decision as well. The upshot, in both my view and that of the PC, is that mandatory vetting, either by judicial or quasi-judicial review, will complicate the procedure of arriving at decisions without providing better ones.[10] We should thus leave the decision up to the family and physician, relying on the concurrence of the latter as a hedge against the ill-judgment of the former, and conscientiousness and the fear of legal action as a sufficient safeguard against that of the latter.

It is not clear to what extent the CLRC agrees and disagrees with these recommendations. While it clearly rejects the idea of mandatory review of any sort, it gives a nominally different answer to the "Who is to decide?" question in its Final Report, claiming that the decision is ultimately up to the physician (26). That sounds like disagreement. On the other hand, it also insists that the decision should be made only after consultation with the family (26), and this sounds like agreement. Consultation is one thing, however, and final say quite another: the fact that the CLRC, in contrast to the PC, recommends that the physician alone should bear full legal responsibility for such decisions lends weight to the view that it thinks he should have the dominant say.

But if the CLRC does think this – and whether it does or not is never made perfectly clear – it is wrong. Certainly in cases of dispute where there is no urgency about the decision, the matter should be (as the CLRC recommends) sent to the courts if further consultations cannot resolve it. We may also agree that if delay is impossible, and the family says do not treat and the physician disagrees, he should be able to override them. But if the family says treat and the physician disagrees, he should surely not be able to override the family's request. But if not, it is not the physician's judgment to which to ultimate appeal is made, but the principle of protection of life.

If, however, physicians do not have the final say, it is odd to hold them solely responsible at law. If family and physician join in a reckless disregard for life or are otherwise negligent, I cannot see why one party should automatically be exempted from criminal liability. The equal voice view of the right to make decisions entails an equal responsibility view of legal culpability. The CLRC is thus faced with a dilemma. If it holds that physicians bear full responsibility, it is committed to the unacceptable view that the family does not have an equal say in the decision. And if it says that the family is at least an equal partner in the decision, it cannot hew to its position that the physician is solely responsible in the eyes of the law.

In conclusion, the PC's report must be judged superior to that of the CLRC in both the clarity and content of its recommendations. The PC seizes on the principle of self-determination and consistently follows out its implications. The CLRC likewise seizes on that principle, but loses its grip in applying it.

NOTES

1 Law Reform Commission of Canada, *Euthanasia, Aiding Suicide and Cessation of Treatment,* Working paper 28 (Ottawa: Minister of Supply and Services 1982)
2 Law Reform Commission of Canada, *Report on Euthanasia, Aiding Suicide and Cessation of Treatment,* Report 20 (Ottawa: Minister of Supply and Services 1983)
3 President's Commission for the Study of Ethical Problems in Medicine and Biomedical and Behavioral Research, *Deciding to Forgo Life-sustaining Treatment* (Washington, DC: U.S. Government Printing Office 1983)
4 In re *Quinlan,* 70 NJ 10, 355 A. 2d 647, 699, cert. denied, 429 U.S. 922 (1976)
5 *Superintendent of Belchertown State School* v. *Saikewicz,* 370 NE2d 417 434–35 (MA 1977)
6 Re *Stephen Dawson. Supt. of Family and Child Service* v. *Robert Dawson; Pub. Trustee for B.C.* v. *Supt. of Family and Child Service* (SCBC 1983), 42 BCLR 173
7 President's Commission, Appendix D
8 See note 5 above. Charles Baron, "Assuring 'detached but passionate investigation and decision': The role of guardians ad litem in *Saikewicz*-type cases," *American Journal of Law and Medicine,* 4 (1978): 111–30
9 See note 4 above.
10 I have expanded my views on ethics committees in "Ethics committees for what?" *CMAJ,* 136 (1987): 1149–51.

13

Proxy Consent for Research on the Incompetent Elderly

BARRY F. BROWN

In the past decade, the ethical issues of research with the elderly have become of increasing interest in gerontology, medicine, law, and biomedical ethics. In particular, the issue has been raised whether the elderly deserve special protection as a dependent group (Ratzan 1980). One of the most profound difficulties in this area of reflection is that of the justification of proxy consent for research on borderline or definitely incompetent patients.

Some diseases of the elderly, such as Alzheimer's disease, cause senile dementia: devastating for the patient and family and, in future, a considerable burden for society. This condition, in turn, renders a patient incapable of giving informed, voluntary consent to research procedures designed to learn about the natural history of the disease, to control it, and to find a cure. The research must be done on human subjects, since there is not as yet a suitable animal model; indeed some feel that there never can be such a model. A protection of the patient, rooted in concern for his best interests, from procedures to which he cannot give consent gives rise to a paradox: "If we can only perform senile dementia research using demented patients, but should not allow them to participate because they are incompetent, then we are left in a quandary. We cannot ethically conduct senile dementia research using demented patients because they are incompetent; but we cannot technically perform it using competent subjects because they are not demented" (Ratzan 1980: 36). Such a position seems to protect demented patients at the expense of their exposure, as a class, to prolonged misery or death.

If the patient cannot give consent, is the proxy consent of relatives ethically valid? That is, do the relatives have the moral right or capacity to give consent for procedures that may not offer much hope for the patient in that they may not offer a direct benefit to him?

Such procedures have by recent convention been called non-therapeutic. They might offer a possible benefit for other sufferers in the future, but little hope of benefit for *this* patient, here and now.

At present, an impasse has developed regarding such research. It appears that such procedures might be illegal under criminal laws on assault. If the research is strictly non-therapeutic, then no benefit is to be found for the patient-subject. If the requirement of therapeutic experimentation is that a direct, or fairly immediate, improvement in the patient's condition is the sole benefit that could count, then it is difficult to see how this could be discovered. For unlike the case of a curable disease or research on preventive measures for childhood diseases, such as polio, the Alzheimer's patients suffer from a presently terminal illness. Studies of the causation of this condition may hold little or no hope of alleviating the condition in them. There appears to be no present or future benefit directly accruing to them. Others may benefit, but they likely will not. Thus, it seems, there is no benefit in view.

If, in fact, such procedures, even relatively innocuous ones, are illegal, then such research cannot go ahead. If so, such persons will remain "therapeutic orphans" just as surely as infants and children unless proxy consent is valid. If proxy consent is also legally invalid, then the legal challenge to this impasse may be either legislative or judicial. In either case, ethical arguments must be offered as justification for the case that proxy consent is or ought to be legally valid. The following explorations are a contribution to that debate.

Can some kind of benefit for the demented be found in research that offers no immediate hope of improvement? I believe that it can, but the nature of that benefit will be unfamiliar or unacceptable to those who are sure that there are only two mutually exclusive alternatives: a utilitarian conception of the social good pitted against a deontological notion of the individual's rights.

Contemporary biomedical ethics routinely employs three principles in its effort to resolve such dilemmas (Reich 1970; Beauchamp & Childress 1983). These are the principle of beneficence, which demands that we do good and prevent harm; the principle of respect for persons (or the principle of autonomy), from which flows the requirement of informed consent; and the principle of justice, which demands the equitable distribution of the benefits and burdens of research. But the first two obviously conflict with each other in human experimentation: the principle of beneficence, which mandates research to save life and restore health, especially if this is seen as directed to the good of society, is in tension with the principle of respect for persons, which requires us to protect the autonomy of subjects. Moreover, the principle of beneficence requires us not only to benefit persons as patients through research, but also to avoid harming them as research subjects in the process. So there is an internal tension between moral demands created by the same principle. Finally, demented patients are no longer fully or sufficiently autonomous. Standard objections to paternalism do not apply. Consequently paternalism of the parental sort is not inappropriate, but rather necessary in order to protect the interest of the patient.

Simple application of these principles, therefore, will not provide a solution. Underlying the manner in which they are applied are radically different conceptions of the relationship of the individual good to the societal or common good.

In the present framework of philosophical opinion, there appear to be two major positions. On the one hand, some consequentialist arguments for non-therapeutic research justify non-consensual research procedures on the grounds that individual needs are subordinate to the general good conceived as an aggregate of individual goods. This good, that of the society as a whole, can easily be seen to take precedence over that of individuals. This is especially so if the disease being researched is conceptualized as an "enemy" of society. On the other hand, a deontological position argues that the rights of the individual take precedence over any such abstract general good as the advancement of science, the progress of medicine, or the societal good. In this view, to submit an individual incapable of giving or withholding consent to research procedures not for his own direct benefit is to treat him solely as a means, not as an end in himself. In this debate, one side characterizes the general good proposed by the other as much too broad and inimical to human liberty; the other sees the emphasis on individual rights as excessively individualistic or atomistic.

There are strengths and weaknesses in both approaches. The consequentialist rightly insists on a communal good, but justifies too much; the deontologist rightly protects individual interests, but justifies too little. I contend that if we are to resolve the dilemma concerning the incompetent "therapeutic orphan," it is necessary to go between these poles. In order to do so, I wish to draw upon and develop some recent explorations concerning non-therapeutic research with young children. In at least one important respect, that of incompetence, children and the demented are similar. We ought to treat similar cases similarly. I wish also to argue that research ethics requires: (1) a conception of the *common good* that is at once narrower than that of society as a whole and yet transcends immediate benefit to a single individual; and (2) a conception of the common good that sees it not in opposition to the individual good but including it, so that the good is seen as distributed to individuals.

THE LESSON OF RESEARCH WITH CHILDREN

As to the first, we may learn much from the discussions concerning research with children, particularly as they bear upon the distinction between therapeutic and non-therapeutic experimentation. In the 1970s a spirited debate took place between the noted ethicists Paul Ramsey and Richard McCormick on the morality of experimentation with children (Ramsey 1970, 1976, 1977; McCormick 1974, 1976). Ramsey presented a powerful deontological argument against non-therapeutic experimentation with children. Since infants and young children cannot give consent, an essential requirement of the canon of loyalty between researcher and subject, they cannot be subjected ethically to procedures not intended for their own benefit. To do so, he contended, is to treat children solely as means to an end (medical progress), not as ends in themselves (Ramsey 1970).

McCormick, arguing from a natural law position similar to that developed in the next section, argued that since life and health are fundamental natural goods, even children have an obligation to seek to preserve them. Medical research is a necessary condition of ensuring health, and this is a desirable social goal. Consequently children, as members of society, have a duty in social justice to wish to accept their share of the burdens of participating in research that promise benefit to society and is of minimal or no risk. Thus the parents' proxy consent is a reasonable presumption of the child's wishes if he were able to consent (McCormick 1974).

There are two major puzzles generated by this debate over non-therapeutic research in children. First, Ramsey stressed that the condition to which a child may be at risk need not reside within his skin, but could be an epidemic dread disease. Thus, testing of preventive measures such as polio vaccine on children is justified; indeed it counts for Ramsey as therapeutic. This is interesting for several reasons. First, the therapeutic benefit may be indirect or remote, not necessarily immediate. Second, it embodies the concept of a group or population at risk smaller than society as a whole. Third, it apparently allows for considerable risk. There was a risk of contracting polio from the vaccine. Although the risk might have been slight statistically, the potential damage was grave. By Ramsey's own account, a slight risk of grave damage is a grave risk. Thus, he was prepared to go beyond the limit of minimal or no risk on the grounds that the polio vaccine was *therapeutic,* while McCormick attempted to justify *non-therapeutic* research on children, but confined the risk to minimal or none. It is odd that in the subsequent protracted debate, this difference was not contested.

The second major puzzle arises from McCormick's view that fetuses, infants, and children ought to participate in low- or no-risk non-therapeutic research in order to share in the burden of social and medical progress in order that all may prosper. Note that only *burdens* are to be shared, not benefits. This is because the topic by definition was non-therapeutic experimentation. By putting it this way he seemed to many to be subordinating the interests of such subjects to a very broadly construed societal good. But let us remember that the argument for such research in the first place was that without it, infants and children would be "therapeutic orphans." That is, without pediatric research, there could be fewer and slower advances in pediatric therapy.

Although not of direct benefit, such research is intended for the long-term benefit of children, and is thus indirectly or remotely therapeutic. It is not conducted for "the benefit of society" or for "the advancement of medical science"; it is for children in the future. Otherwise, it could be carried out on adults. Thus, such research should be construed as done not in view of broad social benefit but for the benefit of children as a group or a sub-set of society. Of course, if advances are made in medicine for the sake of children, society benefits as well, but this is incidental and unnecessary. The sole justification is provided by the benefits now and to come for *children*. At the same time, such benefits set one of the limits for such research: it should be confined to children's conditions, and should not be directed at conditions for which the research may be done on competent persons.

THE COMMON GOOD OF A DISEASE COMMUNITY

Some of the hints arising from the foregoing debate can now be developed. It is indeed wrong to experiment on an incompetent person for "the benefit of society" if the research is unrelated to that person's disease and he is made a subject simply because he is accessible and unresistant. But is it necessarily unethical to conduct experiments on an incompetent person which attempt to discover the cause of the condition which causes the incompetence, and which may cure it or prevent it in others, even if he will not himself be cured?

In a "third way" of conceptualizing the relation between the individual and the group, the good in view is neither that of society as a whole nor that of a single individual. It involves the group of persons with a condition, such as Alzheimer's disease. Here I turn to a conception of the common good articulated by John Finnis of Oxford. Finnis defines the common good not as the "greatest good for the greatest number" but as "a set of conditions which enables the members of a community to attain for themselves reasonable objectives, or to realize reasonably for themselves the value(s) for the sake of which they have reason to collaborate with each other (positively and/or negatively) in a community" (Finnis 1980: 155).

The community may be either the complete community or the political one, or it may be specialized, such as the medical community, the research community, or the community of children with leukemia, and so on. The common good is thus not the sum total of individual interests, but an ensemble of conditions which enable individuals to pursue their objectives or purposes, which enable them to flourish. The purposes are fundamental human goods: life, health, play, esthetic experience, knowledge, and others. Relevant to this discussion are life, health, especially mental integrity, and the consequent capacity for knowledge, all of which are threatened by diseases which cause dementia.

For my purposes, the community should be considered to be, at a minimum, those suffering from Alzheimer's disease. They have, even if they have never explicitly associated with each other, common values and disvalues: their lost health and the remaining health and vitality they possess. It could be said with McCormick that if they could do so, they would reasonably wish the good of preventing the condition in their relatives and friends.

But the community may be rightly construed more broadly than this. It naturally includes families with whom the patients most closely interact and which interact in voluntary agencies devoted to the condition, the physicians who treat them, the nurses, social workers, and occupational therapists who care for them, and the clinical and basic researchers who are working to understand, arrest, cure, and prevent the disease.

The participation of the patient, especially the demented patient, may be somewhat passive. He is a member of the specialized community by accident, not by choice, unless he has indicated his wish to become a research subject while still competent. Efforts to determine what a demented or retarded person would have wished for himself had he been competent have been made in American court decisions involving an incompetent patient's medical care. These "substituted judgment" approaches may have some worth, especially if the patient had expressed and recorded his wishes while still competent.

An individual might execute a document analogous to a human tissue gift – a sort of pre-dementia gift, in which he would officially and legally offer his person to medical research if and when he became demented. This might alleviate the problem of access to some extent, but it has its own difficulties. A pre-dementia volunteer cannot know in advance what types of research procedures will be developed in future, and so cannot give a truly informed consent except to either very specific procedures now known or to virtually anything. Such a pre-commitment may give some support to the decision to allow him to be a subject. But that decision, I contend, is justified by the claim, if valid, that it is for the common good of the dementia-care-research community, of which he is a member and to which, it is presumed, he would commit himself if he were capable of doing so at the time.

It is true, of course, that one might not ever have wished to participate in research procedures. In this case, the individual should be advised to register his or her objection in advance, along the lines that have been suggested for objection to organ donation in those countries that have a system of presumed consent for such donation. This can be achieved by carrying a card on which such an opt-out is recorded, or by placing one's name on a registry which might be maintained by support organizations. I suggest that unless one opt out in this manner, in the early stages of the disease, he or she be considered to have opted-in. That is, there should be a policy of presumed consent. In any event, as experience with organ retrieval has shown, in the final analysis it is the permission of relatives that is decisive in both those cases in which an individual has consented and those in which he or she has not made his or her wishes known.

The other members of the community may not all know each other. They do, however, have common values and, to a considerable degree, common objectives. There can be a high level of deliberate and active interaction, especially if there is close communication between the researchers, family, and volunteers in the voluntary health agencies.

What, then, is the ensemble of conditions which constitute the common good of the Alzheimer's community? Insofar as the purposes of collaboration include the effort to cure or to alleviate the disease, the common good would embrace, in addition to caring health professionals, a policy of promoting research, its ethical review, a sufficient number of committed clinical and scientific researchers, the requisite physical facilities and funding (some or all of which may be within other communities such as hospitals and medical schools), availability of volunteers for research, an atmosphere of mutual trust between research and subject, and finally ongoing research itself. This list is not exhaustive.

If access to the already demented is not allowed, and if this is essential for research on the disease to continue, it may well be impossible to find the answers to key questions about the disease. The common good of the Alzheimer's community would be damaged or insufficiently promoted. Since the goods of life and mental health are fundamental goods, this insufficiency would be profound.

One essential aspect of this common good is distributive justice. Each patient-subject shares not only in the burdens of research in order that all may prosper, but also the benefits. The benefits are not necessarily improved care or cure for the subject, but generally improved conditions for all such patient-subjects: a more aggressive approach to research, improved knowledge of the disease, increased probabilities for a cure, and others. Since the individual participates wholly in that good, he will be deprived of it in its entirety if it is not pursued. The common good is not so much a quantity of benefits as a quality of existence. It can therefore be distributed in its fullness to each member of the community. So, too, each can suffer its diminution.

Richard McCormick (1974) left his description of the common good unnecessarily broad and sweeping. According to some natural law theorists

(Maritain 1947) the common good is always a distributed good, not simply the sum of parts. It is construed as flowing back upon the individual members of the community, who are not simply parts of a whole but persons, to whom the common good is distributed in its entirety. Thus, not only can the common good of which McCormick speaks be narrowed to that of children as a group (equivalent to Ramsey's population at risk) but the benefits of such research can be seen as redistributed to the individuals of the group. The benefits are not to be taken in the sense of an immediately available therapy, but in the sense of improved general conditions under which a cure, amelioration, or prevention for all is more likely.

CONCLUSION

Some of these observations can now be applied to the case of the elderly demented. First, the debate showed the inadequacy of the simple distinction between therapeutic and non-therapeutic experimentation, which has been challenged on several grounds in past years. For example, May (1976: 83) includes diagnostic and preventive types of research under therapeutic experimentation, whereas Reich (1978: 327) observes that the terms "therapeutic" and "non-therapeutic" are inadequate because they do not seem to include research on diagnostic and preventive techniques. In the area of the development of experimental preventive measures such as vaccines for epidemic diseases, and in the area of diseases in which research is carried out on terminal patients with little or no expectation of immediate benefit for these patients, the distinction is somewhat blurred. In each case, there is a defined population at risk: one without the disease but at great risk of contracting it, the other with a disease but with little hope of benefiting from the research.

Such types of research seem to constitute an intermediate category: the "indirectly therapeutic," involving the hope of either prevention or alleviation or cure. This category as applied to dementia shows some characteristics of therapeutic experimentation in the accepted sense, since it is carried out on persons who are ill and it is directed to their own illness. But it also shares some properties of non-therapeutic research, since it is not for their immediate treatment and, therefore, benefit. The good to be achieved is more remote, both in time and in application, since it is less sharply located in the individual than is therapy as such.

It must be admitted that there is a difference between the testing of a vaccine for prevention of disease in young, healthy children and research on elderly, seriously ill patients. In the former, the child-subjects will benefit if the vaccine is successful, or at least be protected from harm. In the latter, the subjects will not benefit by way of prevention or cure of their disease, but rather simply by being part of a community in which those goals are being actively pursued. The identification of the demented patient's good with that common good is doubtless less concrete than the identification of the child's good with that of his peers. But it seems to me that underlying both these cases is a notion of the common good required to justify all cases of research that do not promise a hope of direct benefit to a person who is, here and now, ill.

Years ago, Hans Jonas (1969) noted that a physician-researcher might put the following question to a dying patient: "There is nothing more I can do for you. But there is something you can do for me. Speaking no longer as your physician but on behalf of medical science, we could learn a great deal about future cases of this kind if you would permit me to perform certain experiments on you. It is understood that you yourself would not benefit from any knowledge we might gain; but future patients would." Although greatly vulnerable and deserving of maximum protection, such a patient might be ethically approached to be a research subject, because the benefits to future patients are in a way a value to him: "At least that residue of identification is left him that it is his own affliction by which he can contribute to the conquest of that affliction, his own kind of suffering which he helps alleviate in others; and so *in a sense it is his own cause*" (Jonas 1969: 532, emphasis mine).

In this case, the individual apprehends a good greater than his personal good, less than that of society: that of his disease class, which is *his* good. Of course, the identification of which Jonas speaks is psychological; he would likely not agree with the approach herein outlined and might require that such participation be through a conscious, free choice of the patient. Nevertheless, it is a real, objective good which justifies his choice and prevents us from asking him to participate in research unrelated to his disease. Can a relative, a son or daughter perhaps, ethically make that decision for an incompetent, demented Alzheimer's patient? If so, it is because, in a sense, it is the patient's cause, the patient's good as a member of a community which justifies that choice. It is not a matter of enforcing a social duty or minimal social obligation here, but seeking a good that lies in the relationship one has to others with the same disease. That same good, as noted above, limits the participation of the subject to research related precisely to his disease, not to anything else.

What is the implication of this for risk and the limits of risk? As has been seen, some wish to allow for exposure of subjects to greater than minimal risk provided only that it is classified as "therapeutic" (though the subjects are not ill). Others, in spite of the fact that the research is intended for the benefit of a group at risk, classify it as non-therapeutic and limit the acceptable risk to minimal levels. Are these the only alternatives? One advisory group has allowed, in the case of the mentally incompetent, for a "minor increase over minimal risk'' in such circumstances (National Commission for the Protection of Human Subjects 1978: 16). This is presumably permitted because the research is "of vital importance for the understanding or amelioration of the type of disorder or condition of the subjects" or "may reasonably be expected to benefit the subjects in future" (17). But what counts as minor increase in risk? Proposed research into Alzheimer's might involve invasive procedures such as brain biopsies, implantation of electrodes, spinal taps, and injections of experimental drugs. Are these of greater risk than that specified by the National Commission simply because they are invasive of the human brain? Or is there clear statistical risk of serious added damage to the brain? These are matters for empirical study. The invasiveness per se should not rule out a procedure. The major limitations should be whether the procedure is painful, causes anxiety, or adds to the already serious damage to the brain. If research involving procedures of greater risk than "minor increase over minimal" is ever to be justified, it must be so by the intent to avert the proportional evils of death or mental incapacity. If these are insufficient, then I fail to see what grounds might be available upon which to base a case for legislative change.

It is clear, then, that should such research be acceptable, it also demands that stringent protective procedures be established in order to ensure that the demented are not drafted into research unrelated to their disease class. This is because the standard, being broader than that of "direct or fairly immediate benefit," is open to an accordionlike expansion, and therefore to abuse. Such safeguards could include: rigorous assurance that the proxy's consent (in reality, simply a permission) is informed and voluntary, the provision of a consent auditor, and various layers of administrative review and monitoring, from a local institutional review board up to a judicial review with a guardian appointed to represent the patient-subject's rights. These procedures may prove to be onerous. But we are on dangerous ground, and as we try to avoid overprotection, which may come at the expense of improved therapy for all, we must also avoid opening up a huge door to exploitation.

REFERENCES

Beauchamp, T.L., & Childress, J.F. (1983). *Principles of Biomedical Ethics*. 2nd ed. New York: Oxford University Press

Finnis, J. (1980). *Natural law and natural rights*. Oxford: Clarendon Press

Jonas, H. (1969). Philosophical reflections on experimenting with human subjects. In T. Beauchamp and L. Walters (Eds.), *Contemporary issues in bioethics*. 2nd ed. Belmont, CA: Wadsworth

Maritain, J. (1947). *The person and the common good.* New York: Charles Scribner's Sons

May, W. (1976). Proxy consent to human experimentation. *Linacre Quarterly, 43,* 73–84

McCormick, R. (1974). Proxy consent in the experimentation situation. *Perspectives in Biology and Medicine, 18,* 2–20

McCormick, R. (1976). "Experimentation in children: sharing in sociality. *Hastings Center Report, 6,* 41–46

National Commission for the Protection of Human Subjects (1978). *Report and recommendations: Research involving those institutionalized as mentally infirm.* Washington, DC

Ramsey, P. (1970). *The patient as person.* New Haven: Yale University Press

Ramsey, P. (1976). The enforcement of morals: Non-Therapeutic research on children. *Hastings Center Report, 4,* 21–30

Ramsey, P. (1977). Children as research subjects: a reply. *Hastings Center Report, 2,* 40–41

Ratzan, R. (1980). "Being old makes you different": The ethics of research with elderly subjects. *Hastings Center Report, 5,* 32–42

Reich, W. (1978). Ethical issues related to research involving elderly subjects. *Gerontologist, 18,* 326–37

14

Gerontology's Challenge from Its Research Population: Updating Research Ethics

BEVERLY BURNSIDE

This paper is based on one that was presented to an interdisciplinary gathering of academics and practitioners interested in ethical issues associated with the study of aging.[1] It was inspired by a newspaper column which had appeared several months previously, written by seniors' advocate Chuck Bayley (1984), who asserted that:

> Seniors must be considered an active part of society and should be involved in matters that affect them. That message was stated clearly at two major conferences sponsored last year by the federal government. The University of B.C., unfortunately, is one of the worst offenders. It has a conference coming up in August on Ethics and Aging that is being discussed by educators, researchers, practitioners and policy makers but not by seniors.

Bayley's comments reflect the opinions of other community seniors who feel that, if research on aging is to be carried out, they, as "experts," should be involved in the process as equals rather than as passive objects. Some go further, questioning gerontology's rationale and the motives of researchers. In this brief paper, I shall discuss a dual ethical issue suggested by the comments of Bayley and others, which may be phrased as follows: *gerontological research, as it is commonly pursued, is unethical because it reflects, and thereby perpetuates, the socially structured inequality of older adults in the wider society*. In other words, an "unethical" procedure takes advantage of an already "unethical" social context. Kelman (1972) has noted that the fact of social inequality between researcher and researched underlies most ethical problems arising in social research. Yet this issue is seldom addressed in standard discussions of "research ethics" (but see Beauchamp et al. 1982).

I shall introduce my discussion with some quotations from Auger's (1983) extensive interviews with community seniors in British Columbia. A participant in UBC's 1982 Summer Program for Seniors asserted: "I know what it means to be old. You can only speculate [which is] a hell of a lot different from my reality of things. And I still pay taxes which means that if I'm going to pay for some of this research stuff they put out I want to know what's going into it and how it will be used" (167).

After attending a meeting of the Canadian Association on Gerontology, one of Auger's "involved" informants reported: "There they all were, the academics, the know-it-all gerontologists. They write these theories about us... I felt I wanted to scream at them: ask me! They don't help us, it's themselves they help... they get the money. I'm damned sick of them putting us in cages. We've got to tell them what we want" (18).

The general attitude expressed by a third individual reflects a widely held point of view: "You can keep your research. Gerontology is like a nasty wart on us, first it took just a little bit of taxpayers' money, now it takes more. It does us no good, you get some experience because you talked with us. Us, we get studied. Doesn't seem fair to me, if they gave us the money to spend on programs and services, instead of giving it to those university people to study and talk, we would all be a lot happier" (101).

These voices join those from other heavily researched groups who have, from time to time, rebelled against their status as "guinea pigs" – native people, blacks, and students, for example. Spokespersons from these groups have charged that in focusing research attention on them, social scientists are placing them in a position where they can be more readily controlled and manipulated in the interests of the existing powers (Kelman 1972). Some researchers agree with this assessment, charging that a latent function of the research enterprise is to perpetuate the social structural status quo, the study of society's deviants and dependents revealing the mechanisms to control them (see Schoepf 1979 for a view from anthropology). Kelman (1972) charges that any study in which psychological or social characteristics of a minority or disadvantaged group are assessed may have damaging consequences for the groups studied. These consequences may stem from the biases that enter in at the point of assessing the characteristics under study, at the point of interpreting the data, or at the point of applying the findings to the formulation or execution of policy. It is frequently noted that such populations are uniquely vulnerable to a blame-the-victim treatment (Ryan, 1971), wherein policies are designed to revamp and revise the researchee, never to change the surrounding circumstances.

The relevance of these issues for aging research has been made clear by Maggie Kuhn (1977):

> Gerontology has assumed the deterioration of the aged and has attempted to describe it in terms which ignore the social and economic factors which in large measure precipitate that deterioration. By reifying the attribute of "old" gerontology reinforces societal attitudes which view older people as stuck in an inevitable chronological destiny of decay and deterioration... when persons who are old, poor, and stigmatized by society become objects of gerontological research they are *seen as problems* by society, rather than as persons experiencing problems created by society [italics mine]. (17)

Just as the medical establishment has tended to regard aging as an illness, social gerontologists tend to view aging as a problem or nexus of problems requiring solutions. Further, problems of aging are generally viewed as deficits in the individual, the existing socio-economic context of aging being taken as a given. Few regard the social system itself as an appropriate target for research on aging, or perceive that social dependency and powerlessness are the source of many "aging problems" commonly attributed to the individual (but see Dowd 1980).

The foregoing discussion suggests that the fact of gerontology's existence in and of itself raises fundamental ethical issues having to do with the social creation of dependent status for a significant segment of society solely on the grounds of age. One of Auger's (1983) informants asserted: "We are a generation used to denials. We have been denied work, a decent place to live if we cannot afford high rents and housing upkeep. We have been denied self-respect and self-worth" (231).

Doing research on aging serves to distance researchers and, by extension, the rest of society, from old age. Objectification of social phenomena and people as "things" is characteristic of positivist research, which cannot proceed except by establishing a basic difference between observed and observer; that is, people who are in some way different from ourselves (Rossie 1973). This differentiating process is not lost on one of Auger's (1983) seniors: "Why do those in the field of gerontology do their research isolated from the input that older people could give? By and large older persons have the gut feeling that they have been viewed as 'sick' persons with needs, or at least the object of concern... there is only one useful answer [to correct this misperception]: more personal contact and sincere dialogue between older persons and the researchers" (165).

Columnist Bayley sums it up: "What my friends object to is the attitude that the seniors are out there and we, the academics, can study them at will and pass some judgement as to what they are like and what is best for them" (personal communication).

This perception is upheld in the comment of one of Auger's (1983) academic informants: "The old cannot be trusted to know what they need; they cannot be objective" (214).

My concern about fundamental ethical issues in research on aging, which developed in the course of research among older adults in the community, led to my involvement in the formulation of ethical guidelines for the recently formed Society for Applied Anthropology in Canada (SAAC). I shall discuss some implications of community seniors' demands for involvement in the research process and show how the SAAC document (1984 draft version) reflects an ideology consistent with these demands. I have neither the space nor the expertise to do justice to all the issues I shall raise. My purpose is to open a discussion on ways gerontologists might begin to democratize research on aging, and to suggest that such a process will enhance the quality of that research.

Anthropological "knowledge" has traditionally been derived from long and intense association with "culture representatives" in an attempt to assimilate their unique worldview. This perspective has generated field methods which are essentially democratic. The relationship between *informant*[2] and researcher is necessarily collaborative, the former being seen as the "expert." Thus, ideally, anthropologists have neither "subjects" nor "interviewees" (Mead 1969, Richardson 1975). Nevertheless, until recently, democracy was not extended further – purposes, processes, and outcomes of research remained inaccessible to the anthropologist's naive informants.

During the decade of the 1960s, anthropologists were forced to respond to demands from increasingly sophisticated study populations for a voice in the research enterprise. Particularly in the case of North American native peoples, failure to anticipate and/or comply with these demands has, in some instances, compromised further research in those locations. Not surprisingly, these embarrassing episodes are seldom reported in the literature. From the perspective of contemporary anthropology, an increasing emphasis on applied research – frequently including advocacy and activism under the rubrics "committed," "action," even "partisan" research (Huizer 1979, Polgar 1979) – has meshed well with a traditional methodology which demanded identification with those being studied. Therefore SAAC's position, stated below, cannot be viewed simply as being reactive to demands from no-long-docile informants. Rather, it reflects the extension of an existing democratic bias in field methods which has embraced virtually all aspects of the research process. The SAAC Guidelines state:

> In general, those from whom information is gathered should be treated with respect and where possible given sufficient information to allow them to participate in the various stages of project development. Particularly where research is related to the concerns of these individuals, their input in formulation, implementation, analysis and publication phases of the project should be sought. When such collaboration occurs the applied anthropologist should ensure appropriate credit as co-author, co-investigator or co-curator.

The notion that the research process can, and should – for both ethical and heuristic reasons – be democratized is certainly not new, nor is it the preserve of anthropologists, although they can, perhaps, claim pioneer status. Sociologist Talcott Parsons (1969) has explored the manner in which achievements in the "professional complex," which includes research, are essentially collective and rely on the contribution of both professional and lay elements. Philosopher Jeffrey Reiman (1979) regards researcher and subject as members of a knowledge-seeking team, each with a special expertise, neither being used simply for the purpose of the other. He points out that the surest sign that a research enterprise is a joint undertaking is that it seeks to produce knowledge of value to all participants, not just to the researcher. Psychologist Herbert Kelman (1972) argues that democratization "would enhance rather than endanger the integrity of social research (and) increase the over-all validity of research products." Nurses Kleiber and Light (1978) urge researchers to consider the practical and ethical advantages of interactive research every time they undertake a new project, suggesting that there are many ways to minimize the professional stance of "objectivity" which places distance between researchers and researched. They ask: to what extent are research procedures dictated by tradition, habit, and, perhaps, personal fears of vulnerability?

Whether or not research can be democratized in more than token ways depends, to a large extent, on the type of research being conducted. This is because the power deficiency of those being researched derives from the structure of that situation itself – although, as has already been noted, low status in the wider society serves to reinforce the imbalance. It is instructive, at this point to look at Cassell's (1980) analysis of variations in power relationships between investigator and those studied in experimental, survey, and field research. Differences in relations between investigators and subjects in various types of research become apparent when they are compared along four dimensions: (1) the relative power of investigators, as perceived by subjects; (2) the control of the setting where research takes place; (3) the control of the research context – how the interaction is designed and defined;

and (4) the direction of research interaction: whether it flows primarily in one direction or two. These dimensions are continua, and the relationships in different types of research vary systematically along them.

Cassell compared four ideal typical forms of research – biomedical, psychological, survey, and fieldwork (participant observation) – on the above dimensions and showed that differences are reflected in the terms used to refer to participants. Table 1 reveals variations in power relationships between investigators and subjects in the four types of research.

TABLE 1: Relations Between Investigator and Subjects*

	Experimentation biomedical	Experimentation psychological	Survey research	Fieldwork (P.O.)
	"subjects"		"respondents"	"informants"
Investigator's power as perceived by Ss	H	H – M	M – L	=
Investigator's control over research setting	H	H	O	negative
Investigator's control over context	H	H	M – L	=
Direction of research interaction	I – S one way	I – S one-way	I – S limited two way	I – S two way

PO – participant observation
I – investigator
S – subject

H – high
M – medium
L – low
O – none

*Varieties of research depicted are ideal/typical types. Actual research projects may differ in many ways (Cassell 1982. Table reprinted with the permission of the American Anthropological Association).

In experimental research, typical in biomedical and psychological studies, power and control are in the hands of the investigators who experiment on *subjects*. In survey research, as practised principally by sociologists, those surveyed are *respondents,* a term connoting the moderate but real power differential that exists in non-reciprocal interrogation. Setting and context are controlled by the investigator but there is limited two-way interaction. Fieldwork, engaged in by anthropologists and some sociologists, is commonly carried out in the context of an egalitarian "participant observation" and those "observed" are traditionally referred to as *informants*. Power is equal and control of the setting is negative, that is, in the hands of informants. Direction of research interaction is two-way.

Cassell's distinctions demonstrate that, since context determines the relationship between researcher and researched, the degree to which the research context is amenable to modification will determine the feasibility of subject participation in each case. Alteration of power relationships will be *difficult*, at best, in experimental research;[3] *feasible* to some degree in survey research; *attainable* in fieldwork. It may be noted here that lack of co-operation among "subjects" will doubtless motivate researchers to increase opportunities for their involvement, even in contexts where true equality is not only unrealistic but undesirable. For example, the sharing of information about the research project would go far to mitigate the structural imbalance in experimental research. Let us now look, necessarily briefly, at the research process in its various stages and consider a partnership of gerontologists and old people.

IDENTIFICATION OF RESEARCH TOPICS

Kelman (1972) has noted that those who sponsor and conduct research are able to define what is problematic. They decide on the questions to be asked and the framework within which the answers are to be organized, thereby determining the range of answers that will be obtained and the uses to which the knowledge potentially can be put. Thus the subjects' power deficiency makes it unlikely that the products of the research will be relevant to their own interests, or will accrue to their benefit.

While it cannot be denied that the political and economic interests of the establishment influence what anthropologists study (via the funding process), they are trained to look to their research populations to identify significant research topics. They take it for granted that meaningful research issues must be derived from the perspective of "insider" knowledge, and strive to transcend their own cultural and subcultural biases, which distort perceptions about what is significant, what is "problematic." Like Gertrude Stein, anthropologists look first not for "the answer" but for "the question."

This approach to social research contrasts sharply with that of gerontology's most influential disciplinary component, normative sociology. Guided by a commitment to the positivist paradigm, traditional sociologists have approached their research populations with ready-made research questions and measuring instruments derived from theories which tend to reflect existing social arrangements and perpetuate stereotypes about the nature of aging. Thus the population to be studied is effectively by-passed as a source of knowledge about the process and meaning of aging. Instead "findings" tend to confirm researchers' assumptions.[4] Having discovered that their methods have not yielded desired enlightenment, some sociologists, in the name of a phenomenological, interactionist methodology, call for gerontological research that "goes into the everyday world of the elderly . . . to observe phenomena which they deem to be relevant to their life situation" (Auger 1983:

31), thus promoting a "radical gerontology" which entertains the possibility that issues deemed important to the old should be included as legitimate concerns of gerontologists (Marshall & Tindale 1978–79). Why is it considered "radical" to ask the old to help identify important directions for aging research? We would do well to accept our "subjects" as colleagues if we wish to address meaningful research questions.[5]

RESEARCH DESIGN AND DETERMINATION OF METHODS

The suggestion that research design and determination of methods involve research populations is a challenging and controversial one. It is important to point out that democratic or participatory research does not necessarily imply complete equality between investigator and subject. Certainly in research design the expertise of the investigator must take precedence over the opinions of lay collaborators. Nevertheless, the investigator cannot disregard the attitudes and concerns of the research population in the design phase of research – let us not forget that the researchee has the power to withdraw. The fact that this power tends not to be exercised by members of powerless groups (Kelman 1972) only increases our ethical responsibility. Design determines method, and research methods reflect the status of "subjects," As Cassell has demonstrated.

SAAC's Ethical Guidelines advocate consultation with research participants to discuss possible risks associated with the use of methods demanded by a particular research design, thus making explicit what is usually glossed over in the consent form. For example, the use of life histories, frequently thought to constitute an ideal research tool in gerontology because of known therapeutic benefits to the elderly, should be viewed with caution if used as a data-gathering device, because guarantees of anonymity may not be justified (cf. Klockars, 1977). In collaborative research, decision making about methods must include those who will be at risk.

Mead (1969) has pointed out that even answering a questionnaire for a mass survey puts the subject in the role of "guinea pig." Kelman (1972) advocates expanding the use of the "elite interview" approach in survey research for the purpose of democratization. This is an approach to interviewing modified for the socially powerful who are seen as "experts" in view of special knowledge and/or experience. They thus become active partners in research and therefore, it is assumed, will be interested personally in the process and outcome.

The evaluative study of the Vancouver Women's Health Collective by Kleiber and Light (1978) is a model of "interactive/open" research which, in fact, began in the "traditional/closed" manner. The transition began to occur when it became apparent that the Collective's philosophy of sharing information and, therefore, power was in conflict with the secretive stance of the researchers, wherein ''objectivity''[6] and ''confidentiality'' were guiding principles. Initially this distance prevented the team of investigators from learning from perceptions of the group. The researchers perceived that, in setting themselves up as experts, they denied that Collective members had a crucial contribution to make in the observation and analysis of their own organization. Information sharing shifted the research process from an external to an internal/external evaluation. Kleiber and Light did use traditional questionnaires and structured interviews, and members co-operated to insure that certain basic standards were maintained, however open these were to discussion. As a way of dealing with change resulting from feedback about research findings, Collective members' responses to these findings were included in the research design.

True collaboration in design formulation is most likely to be realized in so-called ''action research'' (Lewin 1958). It grows out of the needs of a community or group, typically involving a desire for change of some kind. Such a scenario demands that the researcher work closely with those involved, although the potential for full partnership may not always be realized.

DATA COLLECTION

There is a long tradition in anthropology of using ''natives'' as interviewers. While reasons for this were initially linguistic, there is no doubt that the technique increases informant co-operation and enhances the quality of information elicited. Gerontological gossip has it that ''middle-aged'' interviewers are more successful than younger ones – one infers that the use of ''old'' interviewers is seldom considered. An exception is Auger (1983) who reports employing four seniors as interviewers in a questionnaire survey after one female informant asked: ''How hard could it be to ask questions of people, and then repeat what they said. . . if only they [gerontologists] would at least offer to help us learn something from them, it wouldn't seem such a one sided thing'' (166).

If we are willing to train students without prior experience to conduct interviews, why do we not place the same confidence in older adults who are likely to be deeply interested in the research project?

INTERPRETATION OF RESEARCH FINDINGS

The SAAC Guidelines state: ''Findings and their interpretations should be made available to host agencies and communities with opportunity to comment before results of the study are made public.''

Whittaker (1981) points to ''a common discovery in fieldwork experience that those being studied adopt an authoritative perspective on 'how things are' and expect their version to be taken at face value and seriously'' (448). While compliance with such naive expectations is not advocated here, it seems logical to suggest that, in social research in general – and certainly in policy-oriented research – we should ask for ''feedback'' from those studied. Do they agree with the investigator's interpretations, and if not, why not? Huizer (1979) has pointed out that one of the requirements of ''truly scientific'' research is to check one's findings with others in the academic community, usually colleagues. Reporting that he at first wondered why this could not also be done with the people whose lives and problems are being researched, Huizer then turned the question around, querying the scientific value of data about people which have been neither ''falsified'' nor ''verified'' by them.

Accepting that researcher objectivity is a myth, on what basis do we assume that our interpretations are valid and/or that we are competent to exhaust possible alternative interpretations? Whittaker (1981) has noted that the use of interpretive metaphors raises ethical issues not usually acknowledged by researchers. The manner in which findings are ''framed'' may transform research findings in ways that informants might find objectionable – were they privy to these final products. (For example, to paraphrase Whittaker, ''retirees'' are likely to find that they inhabit a ''culture of dependence.'') The sharing of interpretive explanations with informants may enrich investigators' models, or suggest more useful, valid models. Jarvie (1972) has asserted that ''Hubris, pride, the view that we and we alone know, is an attitude incompatible with critical and objective scientific enquiry'' (172). Should we not take seriously the plea reported earlier: ''Ask me!''?

DISSEMINATION OF RESEARCH FINDINGS

The SAAC document states: ''In accord with the Society's objective of stimulating interest and discussion of applied anthropology in Canada the researcher should attempt to translate research projects and disciplinary concerns into lay terms, and to demonstrate their importance to the public. There is, therefore, a responsibility to speak out as educators as well as researchers.'' Not all academics agree with this statement, including, it should be noted, some anthropologists. An unidentified researcher is quoted by Auger (1983): ''Frankly, I don't care whether or not they [the old] understand it or not. . . . I am not interested in collecting data which is useful to them. It must be useful to me. . . and to the scientific community who are my peers'' (213).

But who *is* the research for? We should ask, with Kleiber and Light (1978) where benefits from specific research projects go: ''to the funding body? the researcher's career? the public in general or specific interest groups within the public? members of the researched group?'' (29). These authors suggest that full consideration of who the research is for would help clarify responsibilities with regard to who has the right to know about it. But they are speaking from the perspective of participatory research, which takes for granted the sharing of results. Unfortunately, an honest assessment of ''who the research is for'' would probably do little to alter current practice. Further, since the power imbalance inherent in the research context increases the likelihood that results are irrelevant or even antithetical to the interests of subjects (Kelman 1972) it is small wonder that researchers are not always inclined to ''translate'' their products. Dissemination of research thus appears to be a complex ethical issue involving far more than problems in translation.

Nonetheless, if research results are to be disseminated to the public, translation looms as a primary problem. The use of what is perceived to be unnecessary jargon in social gerontology is probably the most frequently heard complaint from our research population. Although the use of technical terms in the biomedical sciences appears to be at least tolerated and the need for it understood, the function of technical language among social scientists is not so condoned, theirs being the language of everyday discourse. Deloria (1980) has asserted that a balance needs to be achieved between the public's ''right to know'' and the ''tyranny of democratization.'' He suggests that the propensity of the media to reduce complicated theories and studies to the lowest denominator for dissemination places too great a burden on the serious scientific investigator. But if research is likely to be freely reported in the media anyway, it seems particularly important that investigators in esoteric domains provide the ''translations.'' In particular, explanations about ''relevance'' are needed to offset public scepticism about seemingly irrelevant research and demand for ''practical'' studies which will produce immediate results.

Researchers in the field of aging are challenged by the hybrid nature of their audience, consisting as it does of practitioners and seniors as well as academics from many disciplines. The need for summaries of our research in simple language seems obvious. Reports about research in the media attests to the interest of an increasingly educated public; certainly those who do community research in gerontology know that the elderly want to know what is being said about them.

CONCLUSION

The opinions of involved seniors previously quoted clearly articulate a mistrust of academics and their products. Bayley, reacting to an earlier draft of this paper, said, ''At one time I looked upon academics as a source of practical help. Now, I am certain they don't have much to offer; certainly nothing like what can be searched out among older persons." But Kelman (1972) believes that it is self-defeating for those who identify with powerless groups to reject or undermine social research, given its actual and potential contribution to the process of social change, that "organizations representing the interests of the disadvantaged segments of the population must acquire *the capabilities for using research* findings in the development of their own programs and in their inputs to the debate around local and national policies" (1015). The onus is on us gerontologists to demonstrate the value of our research to the elderly. Our task is to change the image of academic gerontology among our critics by making them our colleagues in research.

In summary, I have advocated inclusion of old people as equal partners in gerontological research on ethical, heuristic, and political grounds. I have taken the position that the powerlessness of our research subjects mirrors their status, as a class, in the wider society (cf. Dowd 1980), and that this state of affairs creates a set of extremely complex ethical issues. I have also shown that the research enterprise itself benefits in a number of ways from the process of democratization. But I have also tried to suggest that we may no longer have a choice. Like anthropologists before us, we are being challenged by our research subjects and must learn to work with them if we are to produce meaningful and valid results.

Finally, I have proposed that the orientation of applied anthropology, as reflected in SAAC's 1984 Ethical Guidelines, may be a useful model for gerontologists if reform is undertaken. I conclude with an opinion expressed by one of Auger's (1983) informants: "What they [the old] say and how they say it is a gift to be shared, a privilege that the old person grants to the researcher, not a favour granted to the old by the gerontologists" (273).

NOTES

1 Aging and Ethics Symposium, University of British Columbia, August 1984

2 The terms "consultant" and "co-worker" are now preferred to "informant" by many applied anthropologists and linguists because, like "respondent," "informant" connotes passivity and inequality. In addition, Whittaker (1981) notes that "informant" is "imbued with overtones of stool pigeoning, selling out and other forms of immoralities against one's own peoples," and that the (widely used) phrase "people studied" "suggests the anthropologist's self-consciousness and awkwardness with. . . other possibilities" (439). See Wax (1977) for a further discussion of terminology relating to research subjects.

3 The power of the medical researcher is doubtless greatest vis-à-vis the subject because (s)he draws on both the physician's link to matters of life and death and the mystique

of the "scientist." When carried out in a hospital setting by a white-coated investigator, the institutional aura of legitimacy spreads to the research situation (Kelman 1972).

4 I would nominate Disengagement Theory as the most blatant example in gerontology of the consequences of this methodology. To ask whether or not the elderly "disengage" in a society which institutionalizes mandatory disengagement from the occupational world assumes an ethnocentric acceptance of this institution as "normal" and "right." Further, the "theory" implies that mandatory retirement stems from the needs and desires of older workers and not, as MacDougall has demonstrated elsewhere in this volume, from the needs of economic capitalism.

5 A plea for adopting the perspective of older adults in identifying research issues does not imply uncritical acceptance of all topics thought to be important by seniors. For example, my perception is that activist seniors are preoccupied by a perceived need to improve and expand services for the elderly. If the researcher believes that adding to existing services will perpetuate a dependency model of aging, (s)he will not wish to follow the advice of the research population. Yet this reluctance reflects strong value and belief biases akin to those of the armchair positivist. If we make our biases explicit so that they may be discussed and evaluated along with those of our target population, we may generate truly meaningful research topics (cf. Jarvie 1965; Kleiber & Light 1978).

6 In discussing the "myth of objectivity," Lopate (1979) asserts that recognizing and explaining one's *subjectivity* is a better step toward objectivity than the computer-style version; that failure to take account of one's biases and implicit assumptions stands in the way of achieving the ideal of objectivity.

REFERENCES

Auger, J.A. (1983). Gerontological knowledge and its role in the social production of knowledge. Unpub. PH.D. diss., University of British Columbia

Bayley, C. (1984). Primetime. *Vancouver Sun,* 20 March 1984

Beauchamp, T.L., et al. (1982). *Ethical issues in social science research.* London: Johns Hopkins University Press

Cassell, J. (1980). Ethical principles for conducting fieldwork. *American Anthropologist* 82: 28–31

Deloria, V., Jr., (1979–80). Our new research society: Some warnings for social scientists. *Social Problems* 27 (3): 265–71

Dowd, J.J. (1980). *Stratification among the aged.* Monterey: Brooks/Cole Publishing

Huizer, G. (1979). Anthropology and politics: From naivete toward liberation? In G. Huizer and B. Mannheim (Eds.), *The politics of anthropology.* The Hague: Mouton

Jarvie, I.C. (1965). Limits to functionalism and alternatives to it in anthropology. In D. Martindale (Ed.), *Functionalism in the social sciences.* Philadelphia: Amer. Acad. Soc. & Pol. Science

———. (1972). *Concepts and Society.* London: Routledge & Kegan Paul

Kelman, H.C. (1972). The rights of the subject in social research: An analysis in terms of relative power and legitimacy. *American Psychologist* 27: 989–1015

Kleiber, N., & Light, L. (1978). *Caring for ourselves: An alternative structure.* Vancouver: UBC School of Nursing

Klockars, C.B. (1977). Field ethics for the life history. In R.S. Weppner, (Ed.), *Street ethnography*. Beverly Hills: Sage

Kuhn, M. (1977). Grey Panthers pamphlet distributed at the Annual General Meeting, Gerontological Society, San Francisco, November

Lewin, K. (1958). *Resolving social conflicts*. New York: Harper & Bros.

Lopate, C. (1979). On objectivity in fieldwork. In Huizer & Mannheim (Eds.), *The politics of anthropology*. The Hague: Mouton

Marshall, V.W., & Tindale, J.A. (1978–79). Notes for a radical gerontology. *Int. J. Aging & Human Dev*. 9: 163–69

Mead, M. (1969). Research with human beings: A model derived from anthropological field practice. *Daedalus* 98: 361–86

Parsons, T. (1969). Research with human subjects and the "professional complex." *Daedalus* 98: 325–60

Polgar, S. (1979). From applied to committee anthropology: Disengaging from our colonialist heritage. In Huizer & Mannheim (Eds.), *The politics of anthropology*. The Hague: Mouton

Reiman, J.H. (1979). Research subjects, political subjects, and human subjects. In C.B. Klockars and F.W. O'Connor (Eds.), *Deviance and decency*. Sage Ann. Rev. of Studies of Deviance, vol. 3

Richardson, M. (1975). Anthropologist – the myth teller. *American Ethnologist* 2 (3): 517–33

Rossie, I. (1973). Rossie on epistemological issues in exchange between I.C. Jarvie and Fabian. *Current Anthropology* 14: 320–22

Ryan, W. (1971). Blaming the victim. New World: Pantheon

Schoepf, B.G. (1979). Breaking through the looking glass: The view from below. In Huizer and Mannheim (Eds.) *The politics of anthropology*. The Hague: Mouton

Society for Applied Anthropology in Canada (1984). Ethical guidelines for applied anthropologists in Canada (unpublished working paper)

Wax, M.C. (1977). On fieldworkers and those exposed to fieldwork: Federal regulations and moral issues. *Human Organization* 36: 321–28

Whittaker, E. (1981). Anthropological ethics, fieldwork and epistemological disjunctures. *Phil. Soc. Sci*. 11: 437–51

15

Civil Liberties and the Elderly Patient

ARTHUR SCHAFER

Every year in North America thousands, perhaps tens of thousands, of elderly patients are subjected to involuntary restrictions on their liberty. The restrictions may be physical (for example, locked rooms, jackets, wristlets, or bands) or pharmacological (for example, psychotropic drugs), but in either case they are often experienced as deprivations of liberty.

The justifications usually offered for imposing restraints appeal to the safety of those restrained; they are thought to be "at risk" and require protection from self-inflicted harm. An additional or alternative justification appeals to the need to protect others (patients or medical staff) from harm.

These justifications for restraining elderly patients are sometimes compelling. Nevertheless, the danger of abuse and misuse of restraints is significant and the cost, in terms of individual liberty, is high. It is the principal thesis of this paper that elderly patients are frequently deprived of their liberty illegitimately as a result of the wrong questions being asked, the wrong conceptual model being employed by medical staff and family members. An illustration may help.

THE CASE OF MR. JONES

Mr. Jones is sixty-eight years old and a widower. He is being treated in hospital for a broken hip, sustained as a result of an accident. His injury has healed, and he is ready to be discharged. Mr. Jones lives by himself in an apartment, with occasional assistance from a cleaning woman and a friendly neighbour.

Unfortunately, however, he also suffers from arteriosclerosis, which causes him to undergo periods of confusion. During such periods, he has been found wandering downtown without purpose and at some risk to himself. His children believe that he should not be discharged from hospital to live again on his own. They wish him kept under supervision, either in hospital or in a nursing home.

Mr. Jones, during periods of apparent rationality, indicates that he is aware of his problem and the risks it poses to his health and well-being, but nevertheless he prefers to accept these risks rather than be confined to institutional care. The medical team has decided, in consultation with the family, that Mr. Jones will be confined to hospital until a suitable nursing home place becomes available. They refuse his request to be discharged. When he protests aggressively against their decision, they sedate him to a level that ensures his compliance.

DISCUSSION OF MR. JONES'S CASE

It is important to stress in this case that those who have deprived Mr. Jones of his liberty are motivated by concern for his best interests. Indeed, they do not perceive themselves as depriving him of his liberty. They do not see this because they apply to his case the often paternalistic medical model rather than the civil liberties model. Family and physicians see themselves acting as *parens patriae*. They feel morally justified in sedating Mr. Jones to the point where he loses his freedom of action because they are acting in what they believe to be his best interests, protecting him from the risk of self-inflicted harm at a time when he is presumed to be no longer competent to care for himself.

In the medical model, Mr. Jones is viewed as ill ("demented"). Because he is ill, those who care for him are justified in responding with whatever treatment or therapy seems most likely to promote his welfare. If Mr. Jones is viewed as incompetent, then his protests against this treatment will be dismissed as simply one more symptom confirming his illness. Because the restraints imposed on the patient are regarded as being for his benefit, those who impose these restraints quite naturally feel less inhibition than if they were deliberately imposing some punishment.[1] For example, in a recent case in Quebec, *Institut Philippe Pinel de Montreal* v. *Dion,* the court seems to have assumed incompetence on the basis of Dion's refusal to accept treatment: "The court feels that the respondent's refusal to accept the recommended treatment condemns him to detention in perpetuity and the eventual loss of contact with reality. The court does not believe that a man of healthy mind would do this voluntarily."[2]

The medical model encourages its adherents to take action at the earliest possible moment in order to minimize the possibility of harmful effects. In contrast, the civil liberties model requires its adherents to follow a variety of procedural safeguards when they propose to deprive someone of his freedom. The onus of proof rests with those who would restrict liberty rather than upon the person who is to be deprived of liberty. Insistence upon strict rules of evidence or "proof beyond a reasonable doubt" would, in the medical model, be regarded as erecting unnecessarily cumbersome barriers to the efficient delivery of help to those in need.

The medical model is founded upon compassion and a desire to help, but in practice it may be experienced by the elderly patient as controlling and demeaning. The essence of being a mature adult person is to have others respect one's choices. When an elderly patient is labelled as incapable of rational choice, those who apply the label, as well as others, come to view the patient as not fully a person and, frequently, the patient comes to view himself as less than worthy of respect. In other words, there is a stigma associated with restraints, and the stigma tends to become internalized and so produces a diminution of the patient's sense of self-worth.

MENTAL COMPETENCE

The courts have, in general, established the legal right of a competent patient to refuse treatment, even when the result of such refusal may involve risk of injury or death. The victim of a massive coronary attack, for example, who refuses to take medication or even to alter his work and diet in the face of warnings that such behaviour may be fatal, is recognized as having a right to autonomy which forbids our coercive interference.

In our culture, considerable value is assigned to individual autonomy. We wish to be able to regulate our lives in accordance with principles we have ourselves chosen to accept. We attempt to develop our own conception of "the good life" or "self-fulfillment," and we claim the right to regulate our behaviour with reference to this overall plan so long as this does not involve illegitimate interferences with the plans of others.

Undeniably, the life plans adopted by some people will appear imprudent or foolish to others. Nevertheless, even those who favour a range of paternalistic legislation to protect individuals from self-inflicted harm or foolish decisions concede that a competent adult is entitled to take some risks with his or her life, and even to follow a course of action which may produce serious injury to self. Recognizing someone as a mature adult requires that we respect their right to make mistakes, even serious mistakes which may put their very lives at risk.

Important as respect for the value of individual autonomy may be, it is not an absolute value even with regard to competent adults. Moreover, we often feel justified in interfering paternalistically[3] with the liberty of children on the grounds that they do not yet possess the capacities – intellectual and emotional – required in order to make fully rational and voluntary decisions. Children, especially young children, lack the capacity to formulate life plans and they lack the knowledge and experience of the world necessary to discern and act upon their own rational self-interest. Thus, restrictions upon the liberty of children are justified by the need to assist them in developing the competence necessary for the rational exercise of autonomy.

Paternalistic interference with elderly patients is typically justified by extending the argument as it applies to children: for it is sometimes the case that chronologically mature individuals may lose, either temporarily or permanently, the ability to formulate and carry out life plans or to take rational decisions. If paternalism is permitted or required for children then, by the same reasoning, it must sometimes be permitted or required for adults.

THE CENTRAL ETHICAL DILEMMA

At this point, one is confronted with a serious ethical dilemma for geriatric medicine: in what circumstances is it morally permissible and/or obligatory to restrict the liberty of the elderly patient on paternalistic grounds? When there is a clash between the sometimes competing principles of respect for individual liberty and that of preventing patients from coming to harm, which principle should have priority? What criteria ought to be employed by physicians, nurses, and family members in order to resolve this clash of values?

Many of those who would be horrified by a proposal to use coercion against cardiac patients in order to ensure their compliance with medical recommendations are willing to accept coercion of at-risk elderly patients. The mental confusion experienced periodically by patients such as Mr. Jones will seem a sufficient reason for benevolent compulsion.

One difficulty with this line of reasoning is that caretakers of the elderly may too readily make the leap from "at-risk" behaviour to the conclusion of global mental incompetence, without properly considering all aspects of the situation. Doubtless there are many elderly patients who are completely lacking insight into their condition and who are, in consequence, unable to weigh for themselves the risks and benefits of alternative courses of action. At the same time, however, many other elderly patients have sufficient insight into their condition and sufficient appreciation of their own best interests to be able to decide autonomously which risks are worth taking for which benefits. When medical staff and family ignore the wishes of this second group, thereby depriving them of the right to exercise their autonomy, this constitutes an unwarranted usurpation of civil liberties.

The point which needs stressing in cases such as that of Mr. Jones is that periodic mental confusion, memory lapses, temporary disorientation, and other similar mental deficits are not automatic and decisive proof of global mental incompetence. When an elderly patient suffers from some mild degree of dementia this is not automatic and decisive proof of global mental incompetence. Elderly patients suffering from some mild degree of dementia are not ipso facto incompetent.[4] When a choice has to be made between paternalistic coercion on the one hand and liberty with its attendant risks on the other, those who possess the power to abridge the liberty of the elderly patient have a strong moral obligation to investigate carefully the issue of mental competence.

IDENTIFYING THE MORALLY RELEVANT CRITERIA

Elderly patients are frequently deprived of their liberty illegitimately as a result of failure on the part of family and medical staff to pose the right questions. All too frequently the key normative questions are never explicitly raised because the issue is perceived as a medical rather than a moral problem.

Several important questions need to be explicitly asked and answered before any patient is subjected to benevolent compulsion on paternalistic grounds. Let us consider again the case of Mr. Jones. In his case, some of the relevant questions are: How likely is it that he will come to harm? How likely must it be that he will come to harm in order to justify infringing upon his liberty? How serious must be the predicted harm? How oppressive to the patient is the restriction of his liberty likely to be? How long is it anticipated that the deprivation of liberty will continue? Is there any alternative means available to achieve the desired goal without depriving him of his liberty or without infringing to such an extent upon his autonomy?[5]

Once such questions are raised and openly discussed, a number of guidelines suggest themselves. The less likely the harm, the less serious the harm, the more oppressive the restriction of liberty, and the longer the period of liberty deprivation, the less justified would be the imposition of restrictions. Conversely, the paradigm case for justified use of restrictions would be one in which the risk was very likely, the harm severe, the restrictions necessary for protection of the patient minimal and temporary. The paradigm case of unwarranted restrictions would be one in which the risk of harm was slight, the harm anticipated was trivial, and the restrictions necessary to prevent the harm from occurring were maximally oppressive and long-term.

Moreover, the greater the insight of the patient the less justified would be paternalistic interference. In our case study involving Mr. Jones, one could make a strong argument that Jones's demonstrated rational insight into his condition makes it ethically improper to override his value judgment, even though the risk and the stake may both be significant.

Assessing all the relevant factors in each particular case and factoring in all the morally relevant criteria is a subtle and complex task. Difficult as the task may be, however, it is one which we are ethically and, it can be argued, legally obliged to undertake. It is not adequate to ask simply "is the patient 'at risk'?" or even "does the patient pose a risk of harm to others?"

HARM TO OTHERS

The discussion has to this point been anchored to a case study in which the harm anticipated is to self. Where an elderly patient poses a threat to others (patients or staff), it may be that involuntary confinement will be morally justified by a lower risk and lesser stake than when the risk is only to self. Nevertheless, the questions required by the proposed guidelines are still relevant. The decisions to be made are still fundamentally ethical and value decisions, although they have a medical component. What degree of risk of what degree of harm to others justifies what severity and length of liberty-restriction? Simply labelling a situation as one in which there exists a risk of some harm to others is not an automatic warrant to intervene. The risk may be slight. Or the harm to others may be no more serious than a slight violation of privacy (from a patient who occasionally wanders into the room of other patients or takes off his clothes), or it may consist of verbal abuse directed towards the medical staff. Such disruptive behaviour does pose a problem and should be dealt with, but can it possibly justify heavy sedation or severe incarceration on a permanent basis? The results reported by Dr. Colin Powell et al.[6] confirm strongly the danger of overprediction of danger to self and to others on the part of medical and nursing staff. Since the cost of overprediction is measured in terms of lost liberty and diminished dignity, the burden of proof should rest with those who propose to restrict the liberty of the elderly patient.

Misuse of restraints is most likely to occur when the issues of freedom and coercion are disguised as medical issues. When we employ the civil liberties model, we are compelled to deal explicitly with the relevant moral and value issues. This approach, taken in conjunction with ongoing empirical research into the least restrictive measures available to cope with the problems of harm to self and to others, should lead to a significant reduction in the employment of restraints for elderly patients.

NOTES

1 Morris, H. (1968). Persons and punishment. *The Monist, 52,* 475–501
2 *Institut Philippe Pinel de Montréal* v. *Dion,* CS 438 (1093) 2 DLR (4th) 241, 1983 (transl.)
3 "Paternalism" may be defined as an interference with a person's liberty undertaken primarily with the goal of promoting the welfare of the person being coerced.
4 In the recent landmark case of *Rennie* v. *Klein* (462 F. Suppl. 1131, 1145 [1978]), Judge Brotman of the United States District Court of New Jersey stresses the point that one cannot automatically assume that insane patients ipso facto cease to be competent to give or withhold consent for medication in mental hospitals. *A fortiori,* one ought not to assume that a patient who exhibits symptoms of dementia is necessarily incompetent to give or withhold informed consent to restrictions on liberty. (This case is under appeal.)
5 Dershowitz, Alan (1968). Psychiatry in the legal process: A knife that cuts both ways. *Judicature, 51,* 370–77
6 Powell, C., Mitchell-Pederson, L., Edmund, L., & Fingerote, E. *Freedom from restraint: The consequences of reducing physical restraints in the treatment of elderly persons,* unpublished paper. The proclivity shared by physicians, nurses, and family members of geriatric patients to overpredict danger (to self and to others) doubtless arises, in part, from the fear that if harm does occur, those who failed to take preventive action may be held morally and/or legally culpable. By contrast, when a patient is unnecessarily restrained because of apprehended risk, the erroneous prediction is never vulnerable to falsification.

16

Narrative, Perspective, and Aging

C.G. PRADO

Aging raises numerous ethical issues about prejudicial treatment of the elderly, resource allocation in medical treatment, social responsibilities regarding public- and private-sector pensions, and the like. There are, however, subtler ethical issues that relate less to practicalities and more to quality of life. In what follows I briefly discuss what I think to be the most general of these, namely, the way our lives are negatively affected by the very widespread assumption that advanced age brings with it narrowness of view and inflexibility of response. I also discuss how this assumption may be defeated by a better understanding of certain interpretive tendencies which I believe underlie it.

It is now widely acknowledged that "ageism" is as real as racism and sexism (Levin and Levin 1980). A significant part of ageism is the widespread assumption that narrowed perspectives and decreased adaptive capacity are inherent in advanced age. I will argue that this assumption can be overcome by looking at some narrowing of perspective and decrease in adaptive capacity in a way that detaches them from the question of aging as such.

The aged are commonly seen as a distinct class characterized by health problems, above-average dependency on others, special economic needs, and, most notably, a general decline in competence. Elderly people are perceived primarily as having and posing problems, and only secondarily as competent. Against this, a young or middle-aged person is perceived as primarily competent, and only secondarily handicapped by one or another specific condition. For whatever reasons, our culture casts the aged as a "visible minority" and chronological age becomes a ground for prejudice. I have suggested that a crucial part of this view of the elderly has to do with expectations about their awareness, interests, and adaptive capacities becoming more restricted. Because these expectations are about intellectual capacities, they condition all aspects of interaction between those who hold them and anyone significantly older (Kastenbaum 1964).

But aging is not simply a matter of pervasive and consistent deterioration. A great number of elderly individuals are just so many more competent adults. Admittedly they share problems as a statistical group, but so do adolescents and the middle-aged. Obsessive concerns with perceived personal failure or popularity can be as obtrusive as benign forgetfulness. The problems of the old are simply different; they are not so pervasive and integral to age that they lessen the status of the elderly as human beings.

The specific problem I am addressing is the idea that our intellectual and psychological adaptive capacities decline markedly *as a function of growing older*. The ready diagnosis of senility because of even slightly unexpected behaviour is rarely based on evidence of particular disorders; instead it is an assumption of inexorable growing disorientation and decreasing competence of holistic proportions. As a fifty-year-old academic, I have my forgetfulness taken as a badge of office and not as a bar to abstract thought. But if I were seventy it would automatically be seen as inevitable and a symptom of growing incompetence. Studies do show that the elderly retain less in short-term memory and that their reaction times are somewhat slower in various performance areas, but there is no clear basis for the belief that these differences indicate pervasive and general deterioration (Birren and Schaie 1977). Yet this is precisely what is usually assumed.

Sociologists and psychologists are concerned with the empirical aspects of how the aged are perceived and treated, but there is also need for a philosophical contribution, one that is very general and not tied to particular theories of how we form the specific attitudes that govern our actions. We need a broad conceptual context in which lay persons can examine their own attitudes toward aging and the aged, and in which researchers too can examine their basic presuppositions. Technical data and research on aging unfortunately foster objectification of the elderly as a sort of natural kind, inadvertently further isolating the aged. We need to provide a humanistic framework for the furthering of theoretical and empirical investigation. We need a synoptic understanding of the undeniable changes age brings. This is especially true since prejudicial expectations of perspective narrowness in advanced age do seem to have *some* basis. However, that basis must be understood not in terms of statistics and esoteric research data but in terms of how we deal with experience.

The assumption of perspective narrowness in the aged is probably most evident in the way we patronize the old. It is also evident in the amount of work directed toward defeating that assumption (Henig 1981). Nonetheless, we cannot deny real changes. Not even the most sanguine would claim that advanced age makes *no* difference to our attitudes. I, for one, am not a dualist willing to divorce "the mind" from an increasingly worn body. But some changes, particularly certain attitudinal changes, are not a result of deterioration. My basic point is that we need a new way to think and speak of attitudinal changes that occur as we age, a way that does not yoke those changes merely to chronological aging. Only then can we avoid making the elderly a negatively perceived minority and encouraging gloomy expectations on the part of the young about how they will age.

More specifically, we need a new way of thinking and speaking about attitudinal changes which does not cast individuals of a certain chronological age as inherently problematic *on the basis of age*. But neither should real difficulties be masked by overly optimistic jargon and by stereotypes as dubious as those they replace. A second requirement – and this is the heart of my proposal – is that we be able to describe some attitudinal or perspectival changes as natural developments in how we deal with experience, rather than as being pathological or deteriorative. Aging is a natural process, and some of the changes it brings, even though unfortunate, must be recognized functions of what we *do* as we age, rather than as part of what we become as we grow old. A new way to speak of attitudinal and perspectival change, then, requires that we avoid isolating the elderly in invidious ways, and that we treat the process of aging and some of the changes it brings as being natural as opposed to pathological.

My proposal is made in the context of the rather puzzling tendency to think of aging as *narrowing* perspectives instead of broadening them. In some cultures the aged are valued for their wisdom and experience, but in our technologically oriented culture we seem to consider generations as obsolete as the gadgetry of their time (Neugarten 1968). But my proposal does not attempt to simply reverse matters; it attempts to provide a more generous and productive understanding of age-connected change. It begins with conceptualization of awareness, beyond the most elemental objectification, in narrational terms. That is, once the mass of sensory data we receive is more or less sorted out into so many things and events perceived, the organization of experience should be thought of in terms of the imposition of narrative structures on our awareness. Attitudinal or perspectival change can then be thought of as essentially the imposition of more or less restricted narrative structures. (For related views see, for example, Williams 1986a, b; MacIntyre 1981; Cohler 1981). This basic reconception of the organization of experience as a narrational activity provides the key to understanding how our adaptive capacities may grow more rigid and narrow without attributing that change to deteriorative factors.

I might now articulate a sort of principle: Given the creatures we are, perspective broadness is a fundamental value. To flourish as human beings surely requires that we broaden our perspectives. (We count breadth of perspective precisely as a mark of maturity, yet we perversely deny that breadth to the most mature among us.) Anything that restricts our ability to entertain new concepts, to consider novel possibilities, to understand the unfamiliar, or to rethink the familiar, is bad. Breadth of perspective can be considered otherwise only from the point of view of some single restrictive perspective, such as an obsessive religious or political one. But achievement of perspective broadness is, like fitness, something that requires considerable conscious effort.

It seems that as we grow older and gather more experience our perspectival horizon should broaden. But our negative assumption of perspectival narrowness in the aged runs counter to this. Something comes into play here that I have dubbed "interpretive parsimony," which is perspective narrowness due not to deterioration but rather to economy in how we deal with experience. Interpretive parsimony is basically stereotypic thinking, reliance on favoured constructions, and the tendency to respond to situations as we have responded in the past. The central idea is that economy of construal and response is more of a piece than we generally think, and that it is a function of *training*. We learn to gerrymander experience into familiar shapes, and we get too good at doing so. What we see in many people who happen to be older is the result of inhibitory practices, not symptoms of deterioration due to aging. We see the same thing in younger people, but usually not to so evident a degree simply because they have not had as long to become interpretively parsimonious. What is crucial here, however, is that increase of interpretive parsimony is related to aging only in that as we grow older we pile up experience. Yet interpretive parsimony is usually attributed on the *basis* of age.

As I have argued elsewhere, awareness of the world is best construed in terms of the imposition of organizational structures or scenarios which serve as the bases for action (Prado 1984, 1986). These structures have a reflective integrity and progressiveness which is best captured by thinking of them as narratives, as stories which constitute the perceived world for the individual. In these narratives, what sentience and imagination supply is integrated into sequences, and it is within these sequences that the contents of awareness become things and events – and also within them that we emerge as agents to ourselves (on the role of imagination, see Casey 1976).

There are two points here in need of clarification. First, I am proposing a pragmatic way of thinking and speaking, not pretending to have experimentally discerned actual processes. In this way my narrative proposal is like Freud's psychological dynamic. Second, the imposition of narratives is to be thought of as occurring at a basic, prereflective level, and not as an intentional activity. I am proposing we speak of our coming to be self-conscious agents as occurring within narrative, within stories that shape and define our conscious being. The elements of that defined and shaped being are the differentiated contents of consciousness and the association of those contents with action. I can then say that it appears in reflection that action follows on what are perceived as integrated and progressive sequences, which I am calling narratives. This reflective perception is independent of actual causal processes and provides a basis for discussion of the organization of experience in terms of narratives. The key point is that such organization is an activity which may be engaged in to a more or less permissive degree, as opposed to being a mechanical process that changes only because of causal deterioration. Further, it is an activity that may come to be influenced – to a degree – in a deliberate and reflective manner (Prado 1986, ch. 2).

The suggestion is that the use of narrative, of organizational sequences, begins at an elemental level and progresses until it constitutes interpretation of highly conceptualized experiences by the imposition of ever more complex narratives. But that imposition may grow rigid and parsimonious, overly economical in the use of interpretive structures and their elements. Too few narratives come to be relied on in coping with experiences calling for a broader repertory of construals. What is central here is that the imposition of too few narrative structures will grow more rigid and parsimonious because of *success,* because we manage with a small number of narratives or interpretive structures. In this way, experience and coping with experience do not so much broaden our repertories of interpretive construals as confirm us in a limited number of interpretive practices (Prado 1986, ch. 3).

The advantage to discussing perspective changes as we age in terms of narrative employment is that we can consider the possibility of such changes in a way which relates them to aging innocuously. Perspective narrowing, where it occurs, can be thought of as (sometimes) a consequence of practice and not as a result of deterioration. Dealing with experience must necessarily be a matter of organizing, of paring, of imposing structure. What could be more natural than that we might become too adept at economy?

The trouble is that we have a two-tiered perception of interpretive parsimony. Up to a point we understand that how we deal with experience results in reinforcing certain patterns of thought and behaviour. We are aware of these patterns whenever we consider whether someone who has been engaged in one sort of activity for a long period is competent to engage in another sort. But at some point we begin to see interpretive parsimony as due not to economical interpretive practice but to deterioration of a vague sort, and as precluding productive interaction. We sometimes think in this way of people who have obviously become too set in their ways in connection with an occupation, but we *assume* counterproductive economy on the part of the old. In the case of the elderly, we take parsimony to be a function not of practice but of an inexorable wearing down of the mind and body.

If we come to understand interpretive parsimony as a practical, and not an inevitable, result of chronological age, we are very much less likely to think of the elderly as differentiated by intrinsic characteristics, and we will better understand the naturalness of the process by which interpretive economy becomes counterproductive. But most important, we will be better disposed toward interpretive generosity when we interact with those significantly older than ourselves. We would then see that interpretive parsimony is not always a matter of thinking less well, or just less, because of the sheer weight of years. The consequence is that we will deal with those older than ourselves as full-fledged agents and persons. Not only are we then less likely to treat them in ethically dubious ways in connection with specific matters such as treatment and support, but we are also less likely to objectify them, to treat them as *lesser* persons. In this way the quality of their lives will be improved in a very broad but still ethical dimension.

The general hermeneutical or interpretive problem is one of understanding how meaning is "recognized as such by a subject and transposed into his own system of values and meanings" (Bleicher 1980: 1). Dealing with the aged poses interpretive problems similar to those posed by texts of much earlier times. Certain events, for instance, will be only information to a thirty-year-old but will be constitutive parts of a sixty-year-old's frame of reference. As we must recapture the context of a work distant from us in time, we must sensitively facilitate the provision of a context by the implications of what the elderly say to us – implications that are altogether missed when what they do say is dismissed as somehow faulty. The bulk of the work of entering into an elderly interlocutor's context is understanding interpretive practices which have become integral to his or her way of coping with the world – understanding which is rendered more difficult because these practices are unrecognized *as* practices. Some of a sixty-year-old's behaviour, judgments, and attitudes may appear odd or even bizarre to a thirty-year-old, and that oddness invites the harsh conclusion that the sixty-year-old is not thinking *properly* as opposed to only thinking *differently*. If we always perceive communicative difficulties with the elderly as due to deficiency on their part, rather than to counterproductive interpretive practices, we will objectify them, manipulate them, treat them as something less than persons. We will too easily violate the Kantian ethical imperative that we treat others always as ends in themselves and never as means. We will, for instance, too readily make medical decisions for the elderly without full consultation, assuming their incapacity to fully understand a situation. And that is to behave unethically toward the elderly, albeit with the best intentions.

When we understand that the elderly are the persons they are partly because of interpretive practices they have developed, when we begin with the expectation that misunderstanding is due first to discrepancies of interpretation, to a variety of narrative imposition, we will be more able to communicate successfully. Anything that fails to meet our expectations in what the elderly do and say will then be more carefully assessed; we will try to see what puzzles us as a function of construals different from our own, rather than too quickly assume deficiencies and reduce the person in question from someone with whom we must interact to something with which we must deal. The other side of this coin is that the person in question will sense our efforts and there will be a reciprocal effort to communicate more effectively. Moreover, when the overly parsimonious understand that their counterproductive economy is practical and not inherent, they can see that parsimony as reversible instead of accepting it as an inevitable consequence of aging. The reversal of parsimony may range from personal attempts to be more flexible in dealing with others and with situations, to professionally directed therapy. At one end of the spectrum a person – of any age – can monitor her own reactions to people and events, asking herself if she is not construing what she encounters in too limited a way; at the other end there could be therapies in which individuals are made aware that dealing with anyone or anything always involves interpretation, and then made aware of their own interpretive practices with a view to broadening them (for a sketch of the form such therapies might take, see Prado 1986: 130–35). Even simply learning that one *does* interpret in this way may be therapeutically productive, for it forces individuals to realize that there is an activity in which they unconsciously engage that shapes the world in which they live. Once that is realized, they can set about doing things more productively. In this way, reconception of perspectival narrowing in terms of counterproductive interpretive practices not only rids some of us of prejudicial attitudes, but also offers real hope to those who are the objects of those attitudes.

REFERENCES

Birren, James E., & Schaie, Warner K. (Eds.) (1977). *Handbook of the psychology of aging*. New York: Van Nostrand Reinhold. Especially see part 4.

Bleicher, Josef (1980). *Contemporary hermeneutics*. London: Routledge and Kegan Paul

Casey, Edward (1976). *Imagining*. Bloomington: Indiana University Press

Cohler, Bertram (1981). *Mothers, grandmothers, and daughters: Personality and child care in three-generation families*. New York: Wiley. This is the only book of Cohler's that I have seen, having learned of his work from comments by the reviewers of the articles in this collection. Cohler uses the notion of narrative in understanding human development.

Henig, Robin Marantz (1981). *The myth of senility: Misconceptions about the brain and aging*. New York: Doubleday

Kastenbaum, Robert (Ed.) (1964. *New thoughts on old age*. New York: Springer

Levin, Jack, & Levin, William (1980). *Ageism: Prejudice and discrimination against the elderly*. Belmont, MA: Wadsworth

MacIntyre, Alisdair (1981). *After virtue*. Notre Dame: University of Notre Dame Press, ch. 15

Neugarten, Bernice L. (Ed.) (1968). *Middle age and aging*. Chicago: University of Chicago Press. Especially see appendices A and B.

Prado, C.G. (1984). *Making believe: Philosophical reflections on fiction*. Westport: Greenwood Press

———. (1986). *Rethinking how we age: A new view of the aging mind*. Westport, CT: Greenwood Press

Williams, Gareth (1986). Common-sense beliefs about illness: A mediating role for the doctors. *Lancet*, 20/27 December, 1435–37

———. (1986). Lay beliefs about the causes of rheumatoid arthritis: Their implications for rehabilitation. *International Rehabilitory Medicine*, *8*, 65–68

PART THREE

Bibliography

Bibliography

JAMES E. THORNTON, ANNE D. EVANS, GERRY BATES, AND MEGAN STUART-STUBBS

As the Canadian population ages, complex issues concerning the role, capacity, quality of life, and treatment of the elderly are being encountered. These issues give rise to problems regarding social policy and professional conduct, problems which are essentially those of social morality. In an attempt to resolve these problems and the questions they generate, we must consider economic reality and reasons of expediency. At the same time, we must recognize that moral reasoning and justification must be an integral part of the resolution of any practical problem.

Traditionally, literature dealing with the concerns of the elderly has focused on "practical" solutions to identified problems. Over the past decade there has been a noticeable change in this literature. An increasing number of articles and books have appeared which deal exclusively, or in part, with the ethical aspects of the decisionmaking process. There is, however, no readily available "source document" addressing these complex ethical issues. With this in mind, the following bibliography has been compiled to bring together selected literature from several disciplines and professions. Among these are philosophy, medicine, nursing, social work, law, political economics, and public administration. Since practical and ethical issues cannot be totally separated, selections must deal with the process of aging, practical problems experienced by the elderly, and general ethical issued directly relevant to the aged.

To provide a better understanding of the elderly, literature is cited on general social, psychological, behavioural, and physiological aspects of aging. Citations are included on various paradigms of aging, the effects of ageism, and the complexities of inter-family relationships. Issues of public policy are cited as well as articles and books dealing specifically with guardianship, health care policy, housing, income security, retirement, and the rights of the elderly. Health care is a major concern of older adults and the care-givers who provide it. Advances in medical knowledge and technology have made it possible to provide more effective medical treatment and to postpone the moment of death. At the same time, many health care consumers are demanding more active participation in decisionmaking regarding their medical treatment. Finally, selections are included dealing with autonomy, competency and consent, death and dying, dementia, nursing care, patient's rights, physician-patient relationships, research involving human subjects, and truth-telling.

The bibliography was developed from several computerized online data bases: Social Science Citation Index [SSCI], Arts and Humanities Citation Index [AHCI], Psychological Abstracts, MEDLINE, and BIOETHICSLINE. The key descriptors that produced the bibliography were: ethics; aging; ethics and aging; aged; attitudes towards aging; aging process; elderly; old age; senior citizens; gerontology; geriatrics; and geriatric patients. These searches were completed in 1987. Those who would like to continue to develop a bibliography on ethics and aging would be advised to consult with a research librarian.

It is hoped that this bibliography will provide a base for continued study of ethical issues of aging. Additional references can be found at the end of each chapter in this volume. The citations that follow, however, do not duplicate these.

A new perspective on the health of Canadians: A Working document (1974). Ottawa: Department of National Health and Welfare

Abernethy, V. (1984). Compassion, control, and decisions about competency. *American Journal of Psychiatry, 141*(1), 53–58

Abramson, M. (1983). A model for organizing an ethical analysis of the discharge planning process. *Social Work and Health Care, 9*(1), 45–52

Achslogh, J. (1983). Moral and ethical aspects of surgery in the octogenarian. *Acta Chirurgica Belgica,* Suppl., 90–95

Aging in the eighties: America in transition. Washington: National Council on the Aging, Inc.

Aging in North America: Projections and policies (1981). Washington: National Council on the Aging, Inc.

Annas, G.J. (1973). The patient has rights: How can we protect them? *The Hastings Center Report, 3*(4), 8–9

Annas, G.J. (1981). Termination of life support systems in the elderly: Legal issues: the cases of Brother Fox and Earle Spring. *Journal of Geriatric Psychiatry, 14*(1), 31–43

Annas, G.J., & Glantz, L.H. (1986). The right of elderly patients to refuse life-sustaining treatment. *The Milbank Quarterly, 64*(Suppl. 2), 95–162

Archbold, P.G. (1981). Ethical issues in the selection of a theoretical framework for gerontological nursing research. *Journal of Gerontological Nursing, 7,* 408–411

Areco's quarterly index to periodical literature on aging

Atchley, R.C. (1979). Issues in retirement research. *Gerontologist, 19,* 44–54

Atchley, R.C. (1980). *The social forces in later life: An introduction to social gerontology* (3rd ed.). Belmont, CA: Wadsworth Publishing

Baer, L.S. (1978). *Let the patient decide: A doctor's advice to older persons.* Philadelphia: Westminster Press

Baker, F.M. (1986). Legal issues affecting the older patient. *Hospital and Community Psychiatry, 37*(11), 1091–1093

Baltes, P.B., & Schaie, K.W. (Eds.). (1973). *Life-span developmental psychology: Personality and socialization.* New York: Academic Press

Bandman, E.L., & Bandman, B. (1978). *Bioethics and human rights: A reader for health professionals.* Boston: Little, Brown

Banting, K. (1982). *The welfare state and Canadian federalism.* Kingston & Montreal: McGill-Queen's University Press

Barfield, R.E., & Morgan, J.N. (1978). Trends in satisfaction with retirement. *Gerontologist, 18,* 19–23

Baron, C.H. (1981). Termination of life support systems in the elderly. Discussion: To die before the gods please: Legal issues surrounding euthanasia and the elderly. *Journal of Geriatric Psychiatry, 14*(1), 45–70

Barrow, G.M., & Smith, P.A. (1983). *Aging, the individual, and society* (2nd ed.). New York: West Publishing

Battin, M.P. (1983). The least worst death. *The Hastings Center Report, 13*(2), 13–16

Bayer, R., & Callahan, D. (1985). Medicare reform: Social and ethical perspectives. *Journal of Health Politics, Policy and Law, 10*(3), 533–547

Bayles, M. (1980). *Morality and population policy.* Alabama: University of Alabama Press

Bayles, M. (Ed.) (1977). *Medical treatment of the dying: Moral issues.* Cambridge, MA: Schenkman Publishing

Beauchamp, T.L., & Childress, J.F. (1979). *Principles of biomedical ethics.* New York: Oxford University Press

Beauchamp, T.L., & Walters, L. (Eds.) (1978). *Contemporary issues in bioethics.* Belmont, CA: Wadsworth Publishing

Beck, A.P. (1986). Nursing the aged patient: Ethics, a reflection, a choice. *Krankenpflege, Soins Infirmiers, 79*(3), 89–90

Beck, C.M., & Ferguson, D. (1981). Aged abuse. *Journal of Gerontological Nursing, 7*(6), 333–336

Beck, C.M., & Phillips, L.R. (1984). The unseen abuse: Why financial maltreatment of the elderly goes unrecognized. *Journal of Gerontological Nursing, 10*(12), 26–30

Bedell, S.E., Pelle, D., Maher, P.L., & Cleary, P.D. (1986). Do-not-resuscitate orders for critically ill patients in the hospital: How are they used and what is their impact? *Journal of the American Medical Association, 256*(2), 233–237

Beland, F. (1984). The decision of elderly persons to leave their homes. *Gerontologist, 24*(2), 179–185

Bennett, J.C. (1982). Ethical aspects of aging in America. In *The ethics of aging: Church mission and practice*. Proceedings of a conference held at Pittsburgh Theological Seminary, 13–14 May 1982. Co-sponsored with the Seminary by the Pittsburgh Presbytery and the Presbyterian Association on Aging

Berghorn, F.J., Schafer, D.E., & Associates (1981). *The dynamics of aging: Original essays on the processes and experiences of growing old*. Boulder, CO: Westview Press

Berkowitz, S. (1978). Informed consent, research, and the elderly. *Gerontologist, 18*, 237–243

Bernstein, J.E., & Nelson, F.K. (1975). Medical experimentation in the elderly. *Journal of the American Geriatrics Society, 23*, 327–329

Bexell, G., Norberg, A., & Norberg, B. (1980). Ethical conflicts in the long-term care of aged patients: Analysis of the tube-feeding decision by means of a teleological model. *Ethics in Science and Medicine, 7* 141–145

Binstock, R.H., & Shanas, E. (Eds.) (1976). *Handbook of aging and the social sciences*. Toronto: Van Nostrand Reinhold

Birren, J.E., & Schaie, K.W. (Eds.) (1977). *Handbook of the psychology of aging*. New York: Van Nostrand Reinhold

Birren, J.E., & Sloane, R.B. (Eds.) (1980). *Handbook of mental health and aging*. New York: Springer Publishing

Boettcher, E.G. (1985). Linking the aged to support systems. *Journal of Gerontological Nursing, 11*(3), 27–33

Bosmann, H.B., Kay, J., & Conter, E.A. (1987). Geriatric euthanasia: Attitudes and experiences of health professionals. *Social Psychiatry, 22*(1), 1–4

Bowker, L.H. (1982). *Humanizing institutions for the aged*. Lexington, MA: Lexington Press

Brombers, S., & Cassel, C.K. (1983). Suicide in the elderly: The limits of paternalism. *Journal of the American Geriatrics Society, 31*(11), 698–703

Brown, M.C. (1981). Giving seniors a choice of services and facilities. *Ontario Medial Review, 48*(1), 45–48

Brown, R.N. (1979). *Rights of older persons: The basic ACLU guide to an older person's rights*. New York: Avon Books

Buchanan, A., & Brock, D.W. (1986). Deciding for others. *The Milbank Quarterly, 64*(Suppl. 2), 17–94

Butler, R.N. (1977). Geriatric medicine: Imperatives. *New York State Journal of Medicine, 77,* 1470–1472

Butler, R.N. (1984). Old age: Right to privacy and patient's right to know. *Mount Sinai Journal of Medicine (NY), 51*(1), 86–88

Butler, R.N. (1975). *Why survive?: Being old in America*. New York: Harper and Row

Butler, R.N., & Lewis, M.I. (1982). *Aging and mental health: Positive psychosocial and biomedical approaches*. St. Louis: Mosby

Calabresi, G., & Bobbitt, P. (1978). *Tragic choices: The conflicts society confronts in the allocation of tragically scarce resources*. New York: W.W. Norton & Co.

Calasanti, T.M., & Bonanno, A. (1986). The social creation of dependence, dependency ratios, and the elderly in the United States: A critical analysis, *23*(12), 1229–1236

Canadian governmental report on aging (1982). Ottawa: Government of Canada

Cassel, C.K. (1987). Ethical issues in the emergency care of elderly persons: A framework for decision making. *Mount Sinai Journal of Medicine (NY), 54*(1), 9–13

Cassel, C.K. (1985). Research in nursing homes: Ethical issues. *Journal of the American Geriatrics Society, 33*(11), 795–799

Cassel, C.K. (1987). Informed consent for research in geriatrics: History and concepts. *Journal of the American Geriatrics Society, 35*(6), 542–544

Cassel, C., & Jameton, A.L. (1981). Dementia in the elderly: An analysis of medical responsibility. *Annals of Internal Medicine, 94,* 802–807

Cassell, E.J. (1977). The function of medicine. *The Hastings Center Report, 7*(6), 16–19

Cassem, N.H. (1981). Termination of life support systems in the elderly: Clinical issues. *Journal of Geriatric Psychiatry, 14*(1), 13–21

Champlin, L. (1984). Protecting the older patient from medical quackery. *Geriatrics, 39*(9), 128–130

Chappell, N.L. (1983). Informal support networks among the elderly. *Research on Aging, 5*(1), 77–79

Chappell, N.L., & Penning, M.J. (1979). The trend away from institutionalization: Humanism or economic efficiency? *Research on Aging, 1,* 361–387

Childress, J.F. (1981). *Priorities in biomedical ethics.* Philadelphia: Westminster Press

Childress, J.F. (1984). Ensuring care, respect, and fairness for the elderly. *The Hastings Center Report, 14*(5), 27–31

Christiansen, D. (1974). Dignity in aging. *The Hastings Center Report, 4*(1), 6–8

Clark, R. (Ed.). (1980). *Retirement policy in an aging society.* Durham, NC: Duke University Press

Clatworthy, P. (1983). Focus on the elderly: Empathy for another era. *Nursing Mirror, 157*(9), suppl. xii

Cluff, L.E. (1984). The meaning of being old in America: The responsibilities of the medical profession. *Transactions of the American Clinical and Climatological Association, 96,* 185–193

Cluny, G., & Penin, F. (1983). The future of the aged patient at the end of an acute disease. *Revue de médecine interne, 4*(2), 147–154

Cohen, K.P. (1979). *Hospice: Prescription for terminal care.* Germantown MD: Aspen Systems Corp.

Cohler, B.J. (1983). Autonomy and interdependence in the family of adulthood: A psychological perspective. *Gerontologist, 23,* 33–39

Cole, T.R. (1983). The "enlightened" view of aging: Victorian morality in a new key. *The Hastings Center Report, 13*(3), 34–40

Corr, C.A., & Corr, D.M. (Eds.) (1983). *Hospice care: Principles and practice.* New York: Springer Publishing

Couchiching Institute on Public Affairs (1979). *Young-old: A North American phenomenon.* Toronto: Couchiching Institute on Public Affairs

Craig, T.J. (1982). Ethical aspects of primary preventative measures among the institutionalized elderly. *Journal of the American Geriatrics Society, 30*(7), 475–476

Cranford, R.E., & Ashley, B.Z. (1986). Ethical and legal aspects of dementia. *Neurologic Clinics, 4*(2), 479–490

Crawford, J. (ed.) (1981). *Canadian gerontological collection III.* Winnipeg: Canadian Association on Gerontology

Cruikshank, N.H. (1980). Some economic aspects of an aging society. *Journal of Health and Human Resources Administration, 2*(3), 355–363

Curtin, L., & Flaherty, M.J. (1982). *Nursing ethics: Theories and pragmatics.* Bowie, MD: Robert J. Brady

Daniels, E. (1985). The elderly: Trapped in the caring net. *Community Outlook,* 13 Feb., 22–24

Davis, J.W., Hoffmaster, B., & Shorten, S. (Eds.), (1977). *Contemporary issues in biomedical ethics*. Clifton, NJ: Humana Press

Denham, M. (1984). Focus on the elderly: ethics of research. *Nurses' Mirror, 158*(3), 36–38

Denham, M.J. (1984). The ethics of research in the elderly. *Age and Ageing, 13*(6), 321–327

Denton, F.T., & Spencer, B.G. (1983). Population aging and future health costs in Canada. *Canadian Public Policy, 9,* 155–163

Denton, F.T., Kliman, M.L., & Spencer, B.G. (1981). *Pensions and the economic security of the elderly*. Montreal: C.D. Howe Institute

Dervin, J., Dervin, P., & Jonsen, A.R. (1981). Ethical considerations in eldercare. In M. O'Hara-Devereaux, L.H. Andrus, & C.D. Scott (Eds.), *Eldercare: A practical guide to clinical geriatrics* (pp. 15–29). New York: Grune & Stratton

Dickens, B.M. (1974). Information for consent in human experimentation. *University of Toronto Law Journal, 24,* 381–410

Dickens, B.M. (1975). What is a medical experiment? *Canadian Medical Association Journal, 113,* 635–639

Dolinsky, E.H. (1984). Infantilization of the elderly: An area for nursing research. *Journal of Gerontological Nursing, 10*(9), 12–19

Dowd, J.J. (1984). Beneficence and the aged. *Journal of Gerontology, 39*(1), 102–108

Dunlop, D.P. (1979). *Mandatory retirement policy: A human rights dilemma?* Ottawa: Conference Board in Canada

Dustan, H.P., Hamilton, M.P., McCullough, L., & Page, L.B. (1987). Sociopolitical and ethical considerations in the treatment of cardiovascular disease in the elderly. *Journal of the American College of Cardiology, 10*(2 Suppl. A), 14A–17A

Dworkin, R. (1977). *Taking rights seriously*. London: Duckworth

Ebersole, P., & Hess, P. (1981). *Toward healthy aging: Human needs and nursing response*. St. Louis: C.V. Mosby

Eggers, J.E. (1985). Elder abuse identified as nursing challenge. *New Jersey Nurse, 15*(2), 20

Eisdorfer, C., & Lawton, M.P. (Eds.) (1973). *The psychology of adult development and aging*. Washington: American Psychological Association

Elder, G. (1979). *The alienated: Growing old today*. London: Writers and Readers Publishing Cooperative

Ellin, J.S. (1981). Lying and deception: The solution to a dilemma in medical ethics. *Westminster Institute Review, 1*(2), 3–6

Englehardt, H.T., & Callahan, D. (Eds.) (1976). *Science, ethics and medicine*. Hastings-on-Hudson, NY: Hastings Center, Institute of Society, Ethics and the Life Sciences

Estes, C.L. (1979). *The aging enterprise*. San Francisco: Jossey-Bass

Estes, C.L. (1986). The aging enterprise: In whose interests? *International Journal of Health Services, 16*(2), 243–251

Ethics and social inquiry (1983). *The Hastings Center Report, 13*(1)

Etzioni, A. (1976). Old people and public policy. *Social Policy*. *7*(3), 21–29

Evans, K.G. (1981). "No resuscitation" orders: An emerging consensus. *Canadian Medical Association Journal, 125*, 892–896

Evans, R.G. (1985). Illusions of necessity: Evading responsibility for choice in health care. *Journal of Health Politics, Policy and Law, 10*(3), 439–467

Evers, H.K. (1981). Multidisciplinary teams in geriatric wards: Myth or reality? *Journal of Advanced Nursing, 6*(3), 205–214

Exton-Smith, A.N., & Evans. J.G. (1977). *Care of the elderly: Meeting the challenge of dependency*. London: Academic Press

Finch, C.E., & Hayflick, L. (Eds.) (1977). *Handbook of the biology of aging*. New York: Van Nostrand Reinhold

Fischer, D.H. (1977). *Growing old in America: The Bland-Lee lectures delivered at Clark University*. New York: Oxford University Press

Fisher, R.H., & Shedletsky, R. (1979). A retrospective study of terminal care of hospitalized elderly. *Essence, 3*(2), 91–100

Fletcher, John (1973). Realities of patient consent to medical research. *The Hastings Center Studies, 1*(1), 39–49

Fletcher, Joseph (1979). *Essays in biomedical ethics*. Buffalo, NY: Prometheus Books

Foner, N. (1985). Old and frail and everywhere unequal. *The Hastings Center Report, 15*(2), 27–31

Foundations for gerontological education: A collaborative project of the Gerontological Society and the Association of Gerontology in Higher Education (1980). *The Gerontologist, 20*(3), Part 2

Freedman, B. (1975). A moral theory of informed consent. *The Hastings Center Report, 5*(4), 32–39

Freedman, M.L. (1985). Medical education in geriatrics: Ethical and social concerns. *Bulletin of the New York Academy of Medicine, 61*(6), 501–505

Fulmer, T. (1982). Elder abuse detection and reporting. *Massachusetts Nurse, 52*(5), 10–12

Fulmer, T.T. (1981). Termination of life support systems in the elderly. Discussion: The registered nurse's role. *Journal of Geriatric Psychiatry, 14*(1), 23–30

Gadow, S. (1979). Advocacy nursing and new meanings of aging. *Nursing Clinics of North America, 14*(1), 81–91

Gadow, S. (1980). Caring for the dying: Advocacy or paternalism. *Death Education, 3,* 387–398

Gadow, S. (1980). Medicine, ethics, and the elderly. *The Gerontologist, 20*(6), 680–685

Gadow, S. (1983, October). Basis for nursing ethics: Paternalism, consumerism, or advocacy? *Hospital Progress,* pp. 62–68, 78

Gasek, G. (Ed.) (1981). *Canadian gerontological collection II*. Winnipeg: Canadian Association on Gerontology

Gaylin, W., Glasser, I., Marcus, S., & Rothman, D. (1978). *Doing good: The limits of benevolence*. New York: Pantheon

Gerontology Research Council of Ontario (1982). *Research issues in aging*. Hamilton: Gerontology Research Council of Ontario

Gibson, D.E. (1984). Hospice: Morality and economics. *Gerontologist, 24,* 4–8

Gilbert, D.A. (1986). The ethics of mandatory elder abuse reporting statutes. *Advances in Nursing Science, 8*(2), 51–62

Giles, J.E. (1983). *Medical ethics: A patient centered approach*. Cambridge, MA: Schenkman Publishing

Gill, D.G., & Ingman, S.R. (1986). Geriatric care and distributive justice: Problems and prospects. *Social Science & Medicine, 23*(12), 1205–1215

Gill, D.G., & Ingman, S.R. (1986). Geriatric care and distributive justice: Cross-national perspectives. *Social Science & Medicine, 23*(12), 1203–1369

Goldman, R. (1981). Ethical confrontations in the incapacitated aged. *Journal of the American Geriatrics Society, 29*(6), 241–245

Goldstein, D.M. (1982). *Bioethics: A guide to information sources*. Detroit: Gale Research

Gordon, M., & Hurowitz, E. (1985). Cardiopulmonary resuscitation in the elderly: Balancing technology with humanity. *Canadian Medical Association Journal, 132*(7), 743–744

Gordon, T.J., Gerjuoy, H., & Anderson, M. (Eds.) (1979). *Life-extending technologies: A technology assessment*. Toronto: Pergamon Press

Graebner, W. (1980). *A history of retirement: The meaning and function of an American institution, 1885–1978*. New Haven, CT: Yale University Press

Gray, J.A. (1980). Do we care too much for our elders? *Lancet, 1*(8181), 1289–1291

Grisez, G.G., & Boyle, J.M., Jr. (1979). *Life and death with liberty and justice: A contribution to the euthanasia debate*. Notre Dame, IN: University of Notre Dame Press

Gross, M.J., & Schwenger, C.W. (1981). *Health care costs for the elderly in Ontario 1976–2026*. Toronto: Ontario Economic Council

Gross, R., Gross, B., & Seidman, S. (Eds.) (1978). *The New old: Struggling for decent aging*. Garden City, NY: Anchor Press

Gryfe, C.I. (1981). Can physicians afford to treat the elderly? *Ontario Medical Review, 48*(1), 17–21

Gunasekera, N.P., Tiller, D.J., Clements, L.T., & Bhattacharya, B.K. (1986). Elderly patients' views on cardiopulmonary resuscitation. *Age and Ageing, 15*(6), 364–368

Gunter, L.M. (1983). Ethical considerations for nursing care of older patients in the acute care setting. *Nursing Clinics of North America, 18*(2), 411–421

Gunter, L.M., Helkman, L.H., Moser, D.H., & Fasano, M.A. (1979). Issues and ethics inherontic nursing. *Journal of Gerontological Nursing, 5*(6), 15–20

Gutheil, T.G., & Applebaum, P.S. (1983). Substituted judgment: Best interests in disguise. *The Hastings Center Report, 13*(3), 8–11

Gutman, G. (Ed.) (1982). *Canada's changing age structure: Implications for the future*. Burnaby, BC: Simon Fraser University Publications

Gwee, A.L. (1981). Professional social responsibility to elders. *Nursing Journal of Singapore, 21*, 32–33

Haber, P.A. (1986). High technology in geriatric care. *Clinics in Geriatric Medicine, 2*(3), 491–500

Hamdy, R.C., & Braverman, A.M. (1980). Ethical conflicts in long-term care of the aged (Letter). *British Medical Journal, 280*(6215), 717

Haney, C.A., & Colson, A.C. (1980). Ethical responsibility in physician-patient communications. *Ethics in Science and Medicine, 7*, 27–36

Hareven, T.K., & Adams, K.J. (Eds.) (1982). *Aging and life course transitions: An interdisciplinary perspective*. New York: Guilford Press

Harris, S.J., Hepburn, J.A., Gray, J.A., Murphy, E., & Carrie, C.T. (1984). What to do with a sick elderly woman who refuses to go to hospital. *British Medical Journal (Clinical Research Ed.), 289*(6456), 1435–1436

Hastings Center Study Group Concerned with Ethics and the Elderly (1984). *Treatment of elderly patients with impaired or diminished competency*. Hastings-on-Hudson, NY: Hastings Center Institute of Society, Ethics and the Life Sciences

Haug, M.R. (Ed.) (1981). *Elderly patients and their doctors*. New York: Springer Publishing

Healy, P. (Ed.) (1981). Issues in medical law in Canada: Special issue. *McGill Law Journal, 2*(4)

Helfand, A.E. (1983). Our responsibility to our aging patients (Editorial). *Journal of the American Podiatry Association, 73*(1), 50–51

Henderson, G. (Ed.) (1981). *Physician-patient communication: Readings and recommendations*. Springfield, IL: Charles C. Thomas

Hermann, H.T. (1984). Ethical dilemmas intrinsic to the care of the elderly demented patient. *Journal of the American Geriatrics Society, 32*(9), 655–656

Herzog, J.P. (1980). *Mandatory retirement in British Columbia: A review of issues, practices and attitudes*. Victoria, BC: Human Rights Commission of British Columbia

Hirschfeld, M.J. (1985). Ethics and care for the elderly. *International Journal of Nursing Studies, 22*(4), 319–328

Hish, D.M. (1987). Planning for decisional incapacity: A neglected area in ethics and aging. *Journal of American Geriatrics Society, 35*(8), 814–820

Hochschild, A.R. (1978). *The unexpected community: Portrait of an old age subculture*. Berkeley: University of California Press

Holzberg, C.S. (1982). Ethnicity and aging: Anthropological perspectives on more than just the minority elderly. *The Gerontologist, 22*(3), 137–142

Howard, J.H., Marshall, J., Rechnitzer, P.A., Cunningham, D.A., & Donner, A. (1982). Adapting to retirement. *Journal of the American Geriatrics Society, 30*(8), 488–500

Howell, M. (1984). Caretakers' views on responsibilities for the care of the demented elderly. *Journal of the American Geriatrics Society, 32*(9), 657–660

Howie, J. (Ed.) (1983). *Ethical principles for social policy*. Carbondale, IL: Southern Illinois University Press

Hudson, R.B. (Ed.) (1981). *The aging in politics: Process and policy*. Springfield, IL: C.C. Thomas

Hurd, M., & Shoven, J.B. (1982). Real income and wealth of the elderly. *American Economic Review, 72,* 314–318

Illsley, R. (1981), Problems of dependency groups: The care of the elderly, the handicapped and the chronically ill. *Society for Science and Medicine, 15*(3, Part 2), 327–332

Ingelfinger, F.J. (1973). Bedside ethics for the hopeless case. *New England Journal of Medicine, 289,* 914–915

Iverson, M. (1980). Who will serve the vulnerable populations?: Human rights and health care for the aged. *Michigan Nurse, 53*(9), 12–13

Jahnisen, D.W., & Schrier, R.W. (1968). Ethical issues in the care of the elderly. *Clinics in Geriatric Medicine, 2*(3), 457–637

Jahnisen, D.W., & Schrier, R.W. (1986). The doctor / patient relationship in geriatric care. *Clinics in Geriatric Medicine, 2*(3), 457–464

Johnson, C.L. (1983). Dyadic family relations and social support. *Gerontologist, 23,* 377–383

Jonsen, A.R., & Butler, L.H. (1975). Public ethics and policy making. *The Hastings Center Report, 5*(4), 19–31

Kalish, R.A. (1975). *Late adulthood: Perspectives on human development.* Monterey, CA: Brooks / Cole Publishing

Kalish, R.A. (1979). The new ageism and the failure models: A polemic. *Gerontologist, 19,* 398–402

Kane, R.L., & Kane, R.A. (Eds.) (1982). *Values and long-term care.* Lexington, MA: Lexington Books

Kane, R., Solomon, D., Beck, J., Keeler, E., & Kane, R. (1980). The future need for geriatric manpower in the United States. *New England Journal of Medicine, 302*(24), 1327–1332

Kapp, M.B. (1982). Promoting the legal rights of older adults. Role of the primary care physician. *Journal of Legal Medicine, 3*(3), 367–412

Kart, C.S. (1981). In the matter of Earle Spring: Some thoughts on one court's approach to senility. *The Gerontologist, 21*(4), 417–423

Katz, J., Capron, A.M., & Glass, E.S. (1972). Some basic questions about human research. *The Hastings Center Report, 2*(6), 1–3

Kayser-Jones, J.S. (1986). Distributive justice and the treatment of acute illness in nursing homes. *Social Science & Medicine, 23*(12), 1279–1286

Kernagan, K. (1982). Politics, public administration and Canada's aging population. *Canadian Public Policy, 8*(1), 69–79

Keyserlingk, E.W. (1979). *Sanctity of life and quality of life.* Ottawa: Law Reform Commission of Canada

Kirchner, M. (1976, 12 July). How far to go prolonging life: One hospital's system. *Medical Economics,* pp. 69–75

Kleinberg, S.J. (1978). The role of the humanities in gerontological research. *Gerontologist, 18,* 574–576

Klopman, T.J. (1985). Experimentation on the elderly patient with cerebral dysfunction: An ethical question. *Special Care in Dentistry, 5*(1), 30–33

Knowles, R.C. (1986). Grow old along with me! *South Dakota Journal of Medicine, 39*(6), 27–32

Kohl, M. (Special Ed.) (1974, July–August). Ethical forum: Beneficent euthanasia. *The Humanist, 34*

Kreps, J.M. (1979). Aging and social policy: The role of the first forum. *Gerontologist, 19,* 340–343

Langslow, A. (1985). Rights and wrongs towards the aged. Part 2. *The Australian Nurses' Journal, 14*(7), 52–54

Lavelle, M.J. (1977, September). An economic analysis of resource allocation for care of the aged. *Hospital Progress,* pp. 99–103

Law Reform Commission of Canada (1981). *Criteria for the determination of death.* Ottawa: The Commission

Law Reform Commission of Canada (1982). *Euthanasia, aiding suicide and cessation of treatment*. Ottawa: The Commission

LaBar, C. (1986). Long term care: Legislation on abuse, neglect and exploitation of the elderly. *Long Term Care Quarterly, 1*(4), i–iv, 1–18

Leivers, S., Serra, P.T., & Watson, J.S. (1986). Religion and visiting hospitalized old people: Sex differences. *Psychological Reports, 58*(3), 705–706

Lentsch, P.M. (1981). Screening of older adults: An ethical issue (Editorial). *Journal of Gerontological Nursing, 7*(4), 215–216

Leonard, L.R. (1982). The ties that bind: Life care contracts and nursing homes. *American Journal of Law and Medicine, 8*(2), 153–173

Levenson, S.A. (1986). Ethical and legal issues in geriatrics: Competence and patient choice. *Maryland Medical Journal, 35*(11), 933–937

Levenson, S.A., List, N.D., & Zaw-Win, B. (1981). Ethical considerations in critical and terminal illness in the elderly. *Journal of the American Geriatrics Society, 29*(12), 563–567

Levin, J., & Levin, W.C. (1980). *Ageism: Prejudice and discrimination against the elderly*. Belmont, CA: Wadsworth Publishing

Levine, N.B., Gendron, C.E., Dastoor, D.P., Poitras, L.R., Sirota, S.E., Barza, S.L., & Davis, J.C. (1984). Existential issues in the management of the demented elderly patient. *American Journal of Psychotherapy, 38*(2), 215–223

Libow, L.S. (1981). The interface of clinical and ethical decisions in the care of the elderly. *Mount Sinai Journal of Medicine (NY), 48*(6), 480–488

Lipsitt, D.R. (1981). Termination of life support systems in the elderly. Introduction: "To be or not to be: decision-making dilemmas in modern medicine." *Journal of Geriatric Psychiatry, 14*(1), 7–12

Lo, B., & Dornbrand, L. (1984). Guiding the hand that feeds: Caring for the demented elderly. *New England Journal of Medicine, 311*(6), 402–404

Lowy, L. (1980). *Social policies and programs on aging: What is and what should be in later years*. Lexington, MA: Lexington Books

Lowy, L. (1983). The older generation: What is due, what is owed? *Social Casework, 64*(6), 371–376

Lusky, R.A. (1986). Anticipating the needs of the U.S. aged in the 21st century: Dilemmas in epidemiology, gerontology, and public policy. *Social Science & Medicine, 23*(12), 1217–1227

Lynn, J. (1986). Ethical issues in caring for elderly residents of nursing homes. *Primary Care, 13*(2), 295–306

Maas, H.S. (1984). *People and contexts: Social development from birth to old age*. Englewood Cliffs, NJ: Prentice-Hall

McCaffery, M. (1979). D. Skelton: Age is not a disease. *Canadian Family Physician, 25,* 353–357

McCormick, R.A. (1978). The quality of life, the sanctity of life. *The Hastings Center Report, 8*(1), 30–36

McCullough, L.B. (1984). Medical care for elderly patients with diminished competence: An ethical analysis. *Journal of the American Geriatrics Society, 32*(2), 150–153

McGhee, J.L. (1983). The vulnerability of elderly consumers. *International Journal of Aging and Human Development, 17*(3), 223–246

McKee, P.L. (Ed.) (1981). *Philosophical foundations of gerontology.* New York: Human Sciences Press

McLaughlin, P. (1979). *Guardianship of the person.* Downsview, Ont.: National Institute on Mental Retardation

McMullin, E. (Ed.) (1978). *Death and decision.* Boulder, CO: Westview Press

McPhail, A., Moore, S., O'Connor, J., & Woodward, C. (1981). One hospital's experience with a "Do not resuscitate" policy. *Canadian Medical Association Journal, 125,* 830–836

McPherson, B.D. (1983). *Aging as a social process.* Toronto: Butterworths

Maguire, D.C. (1974, February). Death, legal and illegal. *Atlantic Monthly,* pp. 72–85

Makarushka, J.L., & McDonald, R.D. (1979). Informed consent, research, and geriatric patients: The responsibility of institutional review committees. *Gerontologist, 19*(1), 61–66.

Mangan, P. (1983). A view on the continuing care of the elderly: The right of choice. *RCN Nursing Standard* (277), 6

Markson, E., & Batra, G.R. (Eds.) (1980). *Public policies for an aging population.* Lexington, MA: Lexington Books

Marsh, F.H. (1986). Refusal of treatment. *Clinics in Geriatric Medicine, 2*(3), 511–520

Marsh, F.H. (1986). Informed consent and the elderly patient. *Clinics in Geriatric Medicine, 2*(3), 501–510

Marshall, V.W. (Ed.) (1980). *Aging in Canada: Social perspectives.* Don Mills, Ont.: Fitzhenry & Whiteside

Mauksch, I.G. (1980). Advocacy or control: Which do we offer the elderly? *Geriatric Nursing (New York), 1*(4), 278

May, W.F. (1982). Who cares for the elderly? *The Hastings Center Report, 12*(6), 32

Medical Research Council of Canada (1978). *Ethical considerations on research involving human subjects.* Ottawa: Medical Research Council

Meier, D.E., & Cassel, C.K. (1983). Euthanasia in old age: A case study and ethical analysis. *Journal of the American Geriatrics Society, 31*(5), 294–298

Meilicke, C.A., & Storch, J.L. (Eds.) (1980). *Perspectives on Canadian health and social services policy: History and emerging trends*. Ann Arbor, MI: Health Administration Press

Meltzer, J., Farrow, F., & Richman, H. (Eds.) (1981). *Policy options in long-term care*. Chicago: University of Chicago Press

Merowitz, M. (1981). Termination of life support systems in the elderly. General discussion: "Company in battle." *Journal of Geriatric Psychiatry, 14*(1), 87–89

Miles, S.H. (1985). The terminally ill elderly: Dealing with the ethics of feeding. *Geriatrics, 40*(5), 112, 115, 118–120

Miller, S.T., Applegate, W.B., & Perry, C. (1985). Clinical trials in elderly persons (Editorial). *Journal of the American Geriatrics Society, 33*(2), 91–92

Minkler, M. (1986). "Generational equity" and the new victim blaming: An emerging public policy issue. *International Journal of Health Services, 16*(4), 539–551

Morganti, J.B., Nehrke, M.F., & Hulicka, I.M. (1980). Resident and staff perceptions of latitude of choice in elderly institutionalized men. *Experimental Aging Research, 6*(4), 367–384

Moses, D.V. (1982). Nursing advocacy for the frail elderly. *Journal of Gerontological Nursing, 8*(3), 144–145

Mulligan, M.A. (1983). Attitudes and humanistic qualities needed in caring for the aged. *NLN Publications* (20–1917), 5–12

National Advisory Council on Aging (1981). *Priorities for action*. Ottawa: National Advisory Council on Aging

Neale, R.E. (1972). A place to live, a place to die. *The Hastings Center Report, 2*(3), 12–14

Neugarten, B.L. (Ed.) (1982). *Age or need?: Public policies for older people*. Beverly Hills: Sage Publications

Neugarten, B.L., & Havighurst, R.J. (Eds.) (1976). *Social policy, social ethics, and the aging society: Conference proceedings*. Chicago: Committee on Human Development, University of Chicago

Newald, J. (1986). Right-to-life issues further clouded by aging population. *Hospitals, 60*(24), 72

Nielsen, K., & Patten, S.C. (Eds.) (1982). New essays in ethics and public policy: Special issue. *Canadian Journal of Philosophy, Suppl. vol. 8*

Norberg, A., Norberg, B., & Bexell, G. (1980). Ethical problems in feeding patients with advanced dementia. *British Medical Journal, 281*(6244), 847–848

Norberg, A., Norberg, B., Gippert, H., & Bexell, G. (1980). Ethical conflicts in long-term care of the aged: Nutritional problems and the patient-care worker relationship. *British Medical Journal, 280*(6211), 377–378

Norman, A.J. (1980). *Rights and risk: A discussion document on civil liberty in old age*. London: National Corporation for the Case of Old People

Nydegger, C.N. (1983). Family ties of the aged in cross-cultural perspective. *Gerontologist, 23,* 26–32

O'Donohue, W.T., Fisher, J.E., & Krasner, L. (1986). Behavior therapy and the elderly: A conceptual and ethical analysis. *International Journal of Aging and Human Development, 23*(1), 1–15

Olson, J. (1981). To treat or to allow to let die: An ethical dilemma in gerontological nursing. *Journal of Gerontological Nursing, 7,* 141–145

Ouslander, J. (1981). Legal and ethical considerations in the care of the elderly (Letter). *New England Journal of Medicine, 304*(7), 428

Palmore, E. (Ed.) (1980). *International handbook on aging: Contemporary developments and research*. Westport, CT: Greenwood Press

Palmore, E. (1981). *Social patterns in normal aging: Findings from the Duke Longitudinal Study*. Durham, NC: Duke University Press

Pearlman, R.A., & Jonsen, A. (1985) The use of quality-of-life considerations in medical decision making. *Journal of the American Geriatrics Society, 33*(5), 344–352

Pearlman, R.A., & Speer Jr., J.B. (1983). Quality-of-life considerations in geriatric care. *Journal of the American Geriatrics Society, 31*(2), 113–120

Pesando, J.E. (1979). *The elimination of mandatory retirement: An economic perspective*. Toronto: Ontario Economic Council

Peterson, D.A., & Bolton, C.R. (1980). *Gerontology instruction in higher education*. New York: Springer Publishing

Petersson, M.M., & Cushen-Morro, B. (1986). Addressing the need of elderly hospitalized patients for conservatorship: A systems approach. *Social Work in Health Care, 12*(2), 61–69

Pinch, W.J. (1985). Ethical dilemmas in nursing: The role of the nurse and perceptions of autonomy. *Journal of Nursing Education, 24*(9), 372–376

Place, L.F., Parker, L., & Berghorn, F.J. (1981). *Aging and the aged: An annotated bibliography and library research guide*. Boulder, CO: Westview Press

Podnieks, E. (1987). The victimization of older persons. *Canadian Journal of Psychiatric Nursing, 28*(1), 6–11

Podnieks, E. (1983). Abuse of the elderly. *Canadian Nurse, 79*(5), 34–35

Poe, W.A. (1980). The physician's dilemma: When to let go. *Forum on Medicine, 3*(3), 163–166

Porter, S. (1985). Ethics and the elderly: Care at what cost? *Ohio State Medical Journal, 81*(6), 400–407

Power, D.J., & Craven, R.F. (1983). ALS and aging: A case study in autonomy and control. *Image: The Journal of Nursing Scholarship, 15*(1), 22–25

President's Commission for the Study of Ethical Problems in Medicine and-Biomedical and Behavioral Research (1983). *Deciding to forego life-sustaining treatment*. Washington, DC: The Commission

Proceedings from the Alberta Symposium on Aging, 1982 (1983). Edmonton, Alta.: Provincial Senior Citizens Advisory Council

Rabkin, M.T., Gillerman, G., & Rice, N.R. (1976). Orders not to resuscitate. *New England Journal of Medicine, 295*, 364–369

Rachels, J. (1975). Active and passive euthanasia. *New England Journal of Medicine, 292*, 78–80

Rango, N. (1985). The nursing home resident with dementia: Clinical care, ethics, and policy implications. *Annals of Internal Medicine, 102*(6), 835–841

Ratzan, R.M. (1980). "Being old makes you different": The ethics of research with elderly subjects. *The Hastings Center Report, 10*(5), 32–42

Ratzan, R.M. (1981). The experiment that wasn't: A case report in clinical research. *Gerontologist, 21*, 297–302

Ratzan, R.M. (1986). Informed consent from the mentally incompetent elderly. *Postgraduate Medicine, 80*(5), 81–88

Regan, J.J. (1985). Process and context: Hidden factors in health care decisions for the elderly. *Law, Medicine, and Health Care, 13*(4), 151–172

Reich, W. (1975). The physicians "duty" to preserve life. *The Hastings Center Report, 5*(2), 14–15

Reich, W.T. (1978). Ethical issues related to research involved elderly subjects. *Gerontologist, 18*, 326–337

Reich, W.T. (1978). *Encyclopedia of bioethics* (4 vols.) New York: Free Press

Reiser. S.J., Dyck, A.J., & Curran, W.J. (eds.) (1977). *Ethics in medicine: Historical perspectives and contemporary concerns*. Cambridge, MA: MIT Press

Retirement without tears: A report of the Special Senate Committee on Retirement Age Policies (1979). Ottawa: The Committee

Rhoads, S.E. (Ed.) (1980). *Valuing life: Public policy dilemmas*. Boulder, CO: Westview Press

Ridler, N.B. (1979). Some economic implications of the projected age structure in Canada. *Canadian Public Policy, 5*, 533–541

Riley, M.W. (1978). Aging, social change, and the power of ideas. *Daedalus, 107*(4), 39–52

Roberts, H.J. (1982). Medical and ethical guidelines for managing the elderly ill (Editorial). *Journal of the Florida Medical Association, 69*(10), 843–844

Robertson, G.S. (1982). Dealing with the brain-damaged old: Dignity before sanctity. *Journal of Medical Ethics, 8*(4), 173–179

Robertson, G.S. (1984). Ethical dilemmas of brain failure in the elderly (Letter). British Medical Journal (Clinical Research Ed.), 288(6415), 486

Robertson, G.S. (1984). Ethical dilemmas of brain failure in the elderly (Letter). *British Medical Journal (Clinical Research Ed.), 288*(6410), 61–63

Robertson, G.S. (1983). Ethical dilemmas of brain failure in the elderly. *British Medical Journal (Clinical Research Ed.), 287*(6407), 1775–1777

Rock Levinson, A.J. (1981). Termination of life support systems in the elderly: Ethical issues. *Journal of Geriatric Psychiatry, 14*(1), 71–85

Rogers, J.C. (1980). Advocacy: The key to assessing the older client. *Journal of Gerontological Nursing, 6*(1), 33–36

Rose, A. (1981). *Canadian housing policies (1935–1980)*. Toronto: Butterworths

Rosenfeld, A. (1976). *Prolongevity*. New York: Knopf

Rosenfeld, S. (1982). O'Bannon v. Town Court Nursing Center: Patients' right to participate in nursing home decertification. *American Journal of Law and Medicine, 7*(4), 469–492

Rosoff, A.J., & Gottlieb, G.L. (1987). Preserving personal autonomy for the elderly: Competency, guardianship, and Alzheimer's disease. *Journal of Legal Medicine, 8*(1), 1–47

Roy, D. (1981). The ethics of biomedicine. *Canadian medical Association Journal, 125*, 689–692

Roy, D.J. (1978). Biomedical developments and the public responsibility of philosophy. In J.W. Davis, B. Hoffmaster, & S. Shorten (Eds.), *Contemporary issues in biomedical ethics* (pp. 277–295). Clifton, NJ: Humana Press

Royal Commission on the Status of Pensions (1980). *Summary report: A plan for the future*. Toronto: The Commission

Rozovsky, L.E. (1980). *The Canadian patient's book of rights*. Garden City, NY: Doubleday

Rybash, J.M., Hoyer, W.J., & Roodin, P.A. (1983–84). Responses to moral dilemmas involving self versus others. *International Journal of Aging and Human Development, 18*(1), 73–77

Ryden, M.B. (1985). Environmental support for autonomy in the institutionalized elderly. *Research in Nursing and Health, 8*(4), 363–371

Saskatchewan Human Rights Commission (1980). Compulsory retirement: Elements of the debate. *Saskatchewan Human Rights Commission Newsletter, 9*(3), 179–193

Saunders, C., Summers, D.H., & Teller, N. (Eds.) (1981). *Hospice: The living idea*. Philadelphia: W.B. Saunders

Schafer, A. (1985). Restraints and the elderly: When safety and autonomy conflict. *Canadian Medical Association Journal, 132*(11), 1257–1260

Schen, R.J. (1985). Misplacement of the elderly in chronic care institutions: Medical, legal and ethical aspects. *Medicine and Law, 4*(4), 385–388

Schost, B., & Sadavoy, J. (1987). Assessing the protective service needs of the impaired elderly living in the community. *Canadian Journal of Psychiatry, 32*(3), 179–184

Schwenger, C.W. (1979). The future elderly: Can we afford them? *Health Care, 21*, 36–38

Seltzer, M.M. (Compiler) (1978). *Social problems and the aging: Readings*. Belmont, CA: Wadsworth Publishing

Shanas, E. (1979). The family as a social support system in old age. *Gerontologist, 19*, 169–174

Shanas, E., & Sussman, M.B. (Eds.) (1977). *Family, bureaucracy, and the elderly*. Durham, NC: Duke University Press

Shannon, T.A. (Ed.)(1981). *Bioethics*. New York: Paulist Press

Shannon, T.A. (1977). What guidance from the guidelines? *The Hastings Center Report, 7*(3), 28–30

Sheldon, M. (1982). Truth telling in medicine. *Journal of the American Medical Association, 247*, 651–654

Siegler, M. (1977). Critical illness: The limits of autonomy. *The Hastings Center Report, 7*(5), 12–15

Skelton, D. (1982). The hospice movement: A human approach to palliative care. *Canadian Medical Association Journal, 126*, 556–558

Slaby, A.E., & Tancredi, L.R. (1977). The economics of moral values: Policy implications. *Journal of Health, Politics, Policy, and Law, 2*, 20–31

Smith, B.K. (1977). *The pursuit of dignity: New living alternatives for the elderly*. Boston: Beacon Press

Smith, M., & Imeson, K.M. (Eds.) (1978). *Law and the elderly: Proceedings of a conference held April 6–8 1978 at the Sheraton Landmark Hotel, Vancouver, B.C.* Vancouver: Legal Publications, Continuing Education Society of BC, Centre for Continuing Education, University of British Columbia

Snow, R.M., & Atwood, K. (1985). Probable death: Perspective of the elderly. *Southern Medical Journal, 78*(7), 851–853

Somerville, M.A. (1979). *Consent to medical care*. Ottawa: Law Reform Commission of Canada

Spiker, S.F. (1978). The role of humanities in geriatric education. *Gerontologist, 18*, 578–580

Spiker, S.F., Woodward, K.M., & Van Tassel, D.D. (Eds.) (1978). *Aging and the elderly: Humanistic perspectives in gerontology.* Atlantic Highlands, NJ: Humanities Press

Spinella, N.A. (1977, July). Update on opposition to death-with-dignity legislation. *Hospital Progress,* pp. 70–72, 81

Staum, M.S., & Larsen, D.E. (Eds.) (1981). *Doctors, patients and society: Power and authority in medical care.* Waterloo, Ont.: Wilfrid Laurier University Press

Storch, J. (1982). *Patients' rights: Ethical and legal issues in health care and nursing.* Toronto: McGraw-Hill Ryerson

Strain, L.A., & Chappell, N.L. (1982). Problems and strategies: Ethical concerns in survey research with the elderly. *Gerontologist,* 1982, *22,* 526–530

Streib, G.F. (1983). The frail elderly: Research dilemmas and research opportunities. *Gerontologist, 23,* 40–44

Struyk, R.J., & Soldo, B.J. (1980). *Improving the elderly's housing: A key to preserving the nation's housing stock and neighborhoods.* Cambridge, MA: Ballinger Publishing

Symposium on social policies for the aging population: Proceedings (1981). Hamilton, Ont.: Office on Aging, School of Social Work, McMaster University

Tancredi, L. (Ed.) (1974). *Ethics of health care.* Washington: National Academy of Sciences

The Gerontologist (1983), *23*(6)

The Hastings Center Studies (1974), *2*(2)

Thomae, H., & Maddox, G.L. (1982). *New perspectives on old age: A message to decision makers.* New York: Springer Publishing

Law Reform Commission of Saskatchewan (1983). *Proposals for a guardianship act. Part I: Personal guardianship.* Saskatoon, Sask.: The Commission

Thomas, J.E. (1986). Indicators of humanhood and the care of aging, chronically ill patients. *Clinics in Geriatric Medicine, 2*(1), 3–15

Thomas, J.E. (Ed.) (1983). *Medical ethics and human life: Doctor, patient and family in the new technology.* Toronto: Samuel Stevens

Thomasma, D.C. (1984). Ethical judgments of quality of life in the care of the aged. *Journal of the American Geriatrics Society, 32*(7), 525–527

Thomasma, D.C. (1984). Freedom, dependency, and the care of the very old. *Journal of the American Geriatrics Society, 32*(12), 906–914

Thomasma, D.C. (1985). Personal autonomy of the elderly in long-term care settings (Editorial). *Journal of the American Geriatrics Society, 33*(4), 225

Thomasma, D.C. (1986). Quality-of-life judgments, treatment decisions, and medical ethics. *Clinics in Geriatric Medicine, 2*(1), 17–27

Thompson, J., Pender, K.K., & Hoffman-Schmitt, J. (1987). Retaining rights of impaired elderly. *Journal of Gerontological Nursing, 13*(3), 20–25

Thornton, J.E. (Ed.) (1984). *Aging as metaphor*. Manuscript submitted for publication

Thornton, J.E. (1984). Issues affecting gerontology education and manpower needs in population aging. *Canadian Journal on Aging, 2*(3), 153–161

Tibbitts, C., Friedsam, H., Kerschner, P., Maddox, G., & McCluskey, H. (1980). *Academic Gerontology: Dilemmas of the 1980's*. Ann Arbor: Institute of Gerontology, University of Michigan

Toward an independent old age: A national plan for research on aging (1982). Washington: National Institute on Aging

Troll, L.E., Miller, S.J., & Atchley, R.C. (1979). *Families in later life*. Belmont, CA: Wadsworth Publishing

Tymchuk, A.J., Ouslander, J.G., & Rader, N. (1986). Informing the elderly: A comparison of four methods. *Journal of the American Geriatrics Society, 34*(11), 818–822

Vander Zyl, S. (1979), Psychosocial theories of aging: Activity, disengagement, and continuity. *Journal of Gerontological Nursing*. *5*(3), 45–47

Veatch, R. (Ed.) (1979) *Life span: Values and life-extending technologies*. San Francisco: Harper & Row

Veatch, R.M. (1972). Models for ethical medicine in a revolutionary age. *The Hastings Center Report, 2*(3), 5–7

Veatch, R.M. (1976). *Death, dying and the biological revolution: Our last quest for responsibility*. New Haven: Yale University Press

Veatch, R.M., & Bok, S. (1978). Truth telling. In W.T. Reich (Ed.), *Encyclopedia of Bioethics* (pp. 1677–1688). New York: Free Press

Veatch, R.M., & Branson, R. (Eds.) (1976). *Ethics and health policy*. Cambridge, MA: Ballinger Publishing

Veatch, R.M., & Sollitto, S. (1973). Human experimentation: The ethical questions persist. *The Hastings Center Report, 3*(3), 1–3

Wakulczyk, G.C. (1982). Respect for the elderly. *Canadian Nurse: Infirmière canadienne, 24*(2), 38–41

Walker, G.K. (1986). Reforming Medicare: The limited framework of political discourse on equity and economy. *Social Science & Medicine, 23*(12), 1237–1250

Wallace, S.E., & Eser, A. (Eds.) (1981). *Suicide and euthanasia: The rights of personhood*. Knoxville: University of Tennessee Press

Walters, L. (Ed.) (1975–1983). *Bibliography of bioethics* (8 vols.). Detroit: Gale Research Co.

Walters, L. (1977). Some ethical issues in research involving human subjects. *Perspectives in Biology and Medicine, 20,* 193–211

Walton, D.N. (1980). *Brain death: Ethical considerations.* West Layfayette, IN: Purdue University

Ward, R.A. (1980). Age and acceptance of euthanasia. *Journal of Gerontology, 35*(3), 421–431

Warren, J.W., Sobal, J., Tenney, J.H., Hoopes, J.M., Damron, D., Levenson, S., DeForse, B.R., & Munchie Jr., H.L. (1986). Informed consent by proxy: An issue in research with elderly patients. *New England Journal of Medicine, 315*(18), 1124–1128

Watts, D.T., & Cassel, C.K. (1984). Extraordinary nutritional support: A case study and ethical analysis. *Journal of the American Geriatrics Society, 32*(3), 237–242

Weeks, J.R., & Cuellar, J.B. (1981). The role of family members in the helping network of older people. *Gerontologist, 21,* 389–394

Weintraub, M. (1984). Ethical concerns and guidelines in research in geriatric pharmacology and therapeutics: Individualization, not codification. *Journal of the American Geriatrics Society, 32*(1), 44–48

Weir, R.F. (Ed.) (1977). *Ethical issues in death and dying.* New York: Columbia University Press

Wertz, R.W. (Ed.) (1973). *Readings on ethical and social issues in biomedicine.* Englewood Cliffs, NJ: Prentice-Hall

Wetle, T. (1985). Ethical issues in long-term care of the aged. *Journal of Geriatric Psychiatry, 18*(1), 63–73

Wigdor, B.T. (Ed.) (n.d.). *Canadian gerontological collection I.* Winnipeg: Canadian Association on Gerontology

Williams, S.E. (1982). Substituted judgment in medical decision making for incompetent persons: in re Storar. *Wisconsin Law Review, 6,* 1173–1198

Wilson, D.L. (1980). Time for a new approach to Canada's older population. *Canadian Medical Association Journal, 122*(7), 829–833

Wilson, S.H. (1978). Nursing home patients' rights: Are they enforceable? *Gerontologist, 18,* 255–261

Wood, J.S. (1986). Nursing home care. *Clinics in Geriatric Medicine, 2*(3), 601–615

Yordi, C.L., & Ross, K.M. (1982). Research and the frail elderly: Ethical and methodological issues in controlled social experiments. *Gerontologist, 22,* 73–77

General Index

aged, the
adaptability, 58–9, 62, 67–8, 73–4, 216–21
as research subjects, 5–6, 12, 183–5, 187–92, 194–7, 200–5
attitudes toward, 5, 7, 12, 21–2, 25–6, 32–3, 39, 42, 61, 67, 77–8, 194–7, 208–11, 215, 220–1
autonomy, 5–6, 9, 11, 19, 22–3, 27–8, 41. *See also* locus of control
cognitive abilities, 12. *See also* cognitive abilities
confinement, 12. *See also* confinement.
demographics, 100–3
dependency, 86, 110–11
dignity of person, 8, 37–9, 45, 84
discrimination, 11, 36, 86, 88, 95, 129–31
education, 47–8, 79. *See also* education
health care, 9. *See also* health care
illnesses, 50, 148–9
income security, 115–17, 136. *See also* income security
individual differences, 65, 67, 77
issues, 4–5, 9
justice, 23–4, 41–2, 48. *See also* justice
responsibilities, 8, 41, 46–7
self-esteem, 25, 67–8, 78
sex differences, 62–3
sexuality, 28
social services, 18. *See also* social services
state of being "at risk," 208–13
values, 64
Age Discrimination in Employment Act (U.S.), 130, 132, 134. *See also* retirement
ageism, 215, 220–1. *See also* aged, attitudes toward
aging
behavioural, 54
biological, 55–6, 59–60, 65
definition, 55, 66
error theory, 56
interdisciplinary approach, 7
models, 33–4, 54–6
myths, 32
normal, 54–6, 67
process of, 9–10, 54–6, 64–7, 76, 217–21
psychological theories, 65
social theories, 78, 194
speed of response, 57
stages, 33–4, 42, 55–6, 66
task complexity, 57
theories, 54–6, 65, 78
allocation of resources, 11, 85, 91, 95, 107, 111, 122. *See also* health care
aged, 34–6
demographics, 114–22
education, 117–18, 120–1
income security, 115–17
individual rights, 23
Alzheimer's disease, 37, 90, 183–4, 187–9, 191–2
anthropology, 197–204
anxiety, 62
artificial feeding, 20, 163–7. *See also* food
artificial life supports, 51. *See also* euthanasia
attention, 58
autobiographies, 68
autonomy, 6. *See also* patient autonomy

"Baby Boomers," 99, 102. *See also* population aging
Barber and Nejdle v. *Superior Court* 2 (California), 167–8

Bégin, M., 137
Beverage Report, 144
bias: definition, 32
Breaker Morant, 39

Canada
  demographics, 85–6, 98–103
  economy, 111
  education, 117–18
  euthanasia, 159–63, 172–9, 181–2
  fertility rates, 100–3
  health care, 10, 116–17, 143–5
  income security, 115–17, 142–4
  labour force, 100–3, 111–14
  pensions, 117–19, 135-40, 142–3
  retirement, 129–36
Canada Assistance Plan, 144
Canada Health Act, 145
Canada Pension Plan, 115, 117, 135, 138–40, 144. *See also* pensions
Canadian Association on Gerontology, 195
Canadian Charter of Rights and Freedoms, 130–1, 134
Canadian Constitution, 27. *See also* individual rights
Canadian Law Reform Commission. *See* Law Reform Commission of Canada
cardiovascular disease
  cognitive abilities, 57
care providers, 18, 81; nursing homes, 80. *See also* family
Cesarec Marke Personality Schedule, 63
children, 43, 47, 68, 78, 88, 110, 210–11. *See also* family, newborns
choices, 18. *See also* ethics, decisionmaking
chronic care, 148–51
cognitive abilities, 56–9, 73–4, 81, 215–21. *See also* memory
  cardiovascular disease, 57
  inactivity, 57
  intellectual stimulation, 57
  socioeconomic status, 57
  terminal decline, 57
common good, 187
communication
  with the aged, 221
community, 36, 187–91. *See also* ethics, values
compensatory strategies, 58–9. *See also* aged, adaptability
competence, 177–82. *See also* confinement, euthanasia
competence, 6. *See also* incompetence
confinement, 208–13
consent: informed, 6, 23; proxy, 183–91
cost-benefit analysis, 23, 91
creativity, 45–6, 67
crisis intervention, 23. *See also* intervention

Dawson v. *Supt. of Family and Child Services,* 173–5
death, 68–9, 160–1, 174
  casual agency, 156–9, 168–70
  locus of control, 19–21, 50–2. *See also* euthanasia
  natural, 56
  with dignity, 36–7
dementia. *See* Alzheimer's disease
demographics, 98–122
  Canada, 85–6, 98–122
  dependency ratios, 86, 107–11
  education, 120–1
  health care, 120–1
  mortality rates, 33–4
  United States, 98–9
Dion v. *Institut Philippe Pinel de Montréal,* 209
disability, 25–6
disengagement, 46
doctor-patient relationship, 38, 148. *See also* physicians
drugs
  aged, 146
  analgesic, 162, 168
  pharmaceutical industry, 148
  sedatives, 209

economics
  demand, 105–11
  demographics, 103–7, 111–14, 122
  dependency, 11
  Gross National Product (GNP), 104–6, 120, 148
  model, 111–14
  pensions, 137–8
  productivity rates, 113, 122
  supply, 105
education, 81, 102, 117–18, 120–1. *See also* aged, education
Elderhostels, 48
employment, 45–6, 130. *See also*

retirement
  labour force, 112
encoding, 57–8, 73. *See also* memory
Epp, J., 137
equality, 84, 87–96, 197–205. *See also* justice
error theory, 56
ethics
  aging, 3–13, 39–40
  biomedical, 12, 86–96, 184–5
  clinical, 31
  confinement, 208–13
  death, 36–7. *See also* euthanasia
  decisionmaking, 18–19, 31
  human capital, 34–5
  income security, 137–8
  intervention, 81–2
  models, 128
  moral reasoning, 3–4
  normative, 4, 10
  pensions, 137–40
  practical, 4
  principles, 9, 184–5
  professional, 17
  purpose, 69
  research subjects, 183–92
  respect for person. *See* aged, dignity of person
  sanctity of human life, 4
  utilitarian, 49, 128
  values, 17, 22–4
ethos: definition, 31
euthanasia, 6, 9, 11, 20–1
  active, 37–9, 51–2, 155–9, 161
  Canada, 159–63, 172–9, 181–2
  incompetence, 177–82
  locus of control, 159, 161, 174–82
  passive, 37–9, 51, 155–9
  physicians' role, 161, 177–82
  United States, 159–63, 172–3, 175–82
evolution: brain development, 65
extra-billing, 84, 145

family
  attitudes of, 25–6
  confining the aged, 209, 212
  consent for research, 191–2
  euthanasia, 179–82
  health care, 151
  housing, 43
  locus of control, 179–82
fertility rates
  Canada, 100–3
  projections, 108–9
food
  meals on wheels, 21
  medical treatment, 20, 164
  symbolic value, 21, 164–7
  withholding, 163–71
freedom, 17, 27, 41–52, 128. *See also* locus of control

gerontology, 65, 78
  attitudes toward, 195–7, 204–5
  ethics, 194–5
  interdisciplinary approach, 7
Guaranteed Income Supplement, 136–40, 144

Hall Report, 84
Hawking, Stephen, 66
health: definition, 150–1
health care
  aged, 34, 106, 117
  allocation of resources, 10, 48–50, 84–96, 116–17, 120–1
  Canada, 10, 44, 84–5, 143–5
  chronic, 148–51
  cost benefit, 23, 89–90
  cost-effectiveness, 90–1
  delivery system, 144, 145–51
  demographics, 120–1
  denial, 86
  drugs, 146. *See also* drugs
  economics, 145, 151
  equity, 23
  ethics, 89–96
  goals, 91
  home care, 147, 150
  hospitals, 145–7
  ideal policy, 93–4
  insurance, 144–6
  medical model, 147–50
  medical profession, 148–50
  prevention, 90, 150–1
  priorities, 150–1
  self-care, 151
  withdrawal, 174–6
hemodialysis, 50, 86
homicide, 167–70. *See also* euthanasia
  Switzerland, 162
hospice movement, 6
Hospital Insurance and Diagnostic

Services Act, 144
housing: retirement community, 42–3
human rights, 12, 27–9, 34, 84, 127–28, 132–40
human tissue gift, 188
hydration. *See also* food, withholding

iatrogenesis, 149
inactivity: cognitive abilities, 57
income security, 11
  Canada, 115–19, 135–40, 142–4
  United States, 43–4
incompetence, 6, 22, 28. *See also* confinement
  diagnosis, 216
  research, 183–91
I Never Sang for My Father, 68
information processing model, 57–8
informed consent, 6, 23. *See also* locus of control
interpretive parsimony, 218–21
intervention, 10, 74–82
  effects, 80–1, 91
  ethics, 75
  goals, 23, 75–8
  rationality, 6
introversion-extroversion, 62

justice, 10, 23–4, 41–2, 48, 142

Kantian ethics, 220
Kafka's Gregor, 25–6

labour force
  Canada, 100–3
  demographics, 105
  rates, 111–14
  retirement, 134–5
Lalonde Report, 84
law
  confinement, 209–10
  ethics, 128
  euthanasia, 11, 161, 172–4, 176–82
  research subjects, 184, 192
  retirement, 129–35
  rights, 27. *See also* individual rights
  treatment, 209–10
Law Reform Commission of Canada, 27, 159–64, 168, 172–8, 181–2
  euthanasia, 160–1
learning, 78–80; models, 57–8
leisure, 46–7
life expectancy, 33–4, 49, 63, 64–5
living wills ("Natural Death Acts"), 6, 11, 51, 161, 176–9
lobbying, 46
locus of control, 76–7, 79. *See also* patient autonomy
  aged, 6
  death, 39
  euthanasia, 11
  research subjects, 183, 186, 188–9, 191, 192, 194–205
loneliness, 21

Manitoba Commission on Compulsory Retirement, 129, 131, 134–5. *See also* retirement
Manitoba Human Rights Act, 132
Manitoba Human Rights Commission, 129
Manitoba Human Rights Commission v. *Finlayson,* 133
Marke Nyman Temperament Scale, 63
Marsh Report, 144
McKinney v. *University of Guelph, 130*
Medical Care Act, 144
medical profession, 19, 38–9, 145, 148–50
  authority of, 38–9
  confining the aged, 209, 211, 213
  euthanasia, 177–82
  values, 81, 174, 208–13, 210
medical technology, 22–23, 35. *See also* biomedical ethics
Medicaid, 44
Medicare, 44
memory, 57–61, 73, 216; types, 57, 60
mortality rates, 33–4. *See also* life expectancy
morbidity model, 33–4

narratives: organization of experience, 218–21
nasogastric tubes, 20, 165
National Commission for the Protection of Human Subjects, 191–2
"Natural Death Acts." *See* living wills
newborns, 38–9, 87–8, 166, 175
nursing homes, 146; dependency, 80

Old Age Assistance Act, 143
Old Age Pensions Act, 142
Old Age Security Act, 115–19, 135, 143

Ontario Human Rights Commission v. *Borough of Etobicoke*, 133
optimum functioning, 77
organ donation, 188–9
organ transplants, 50, 86–7
organization of experience: narratives and, 219–21

paternalism, 6, 210. *See also* locus of control
patient: autonomy, 19, 159, 161, 174–82, 208–13
Pension Benefits Standards Act, 136–7
pensions, 7, 117–19
  Canada, 142–3
  funding, 136–40
  history, 132, 135
  private, 135–8
  Quebec Pension Plan, 115, 135, 138–40, 144
  regressive, 139
perceptual organization, 58
personality, 61–3
  introversion-extroversion, 62
  psychoanalytic theory, 61
  stability, 61–3
politics, 107, 121–2, 137–8. *See also* allocation of resources
  social change, 127
population aging, 98–122. *See also* demographics
poverty, 44, 148. *See also* income security
President's Commission for the Study of Ethical Problems in Medical and Biomedical and Behavioral Research, 86–7, 156, 159–64, 172–80
problem-solving, 58, 60–1
  concept formation, 60–1
  transformation tasks, 60
  psychology, 76–8; theories, 61, 65
  public services, 104, 114–17

quality of life, 76, 91, 160–1, 170, 173–5
Quinlan case (Superior Court of New Jersey), 164, 168–70, 172, 180

rationality: intervention, 6
religion, 47, 51–2, 64, 68–9
research
  common good, 187–92
  consent, 6, 183, 186, 188–92, 201
  democratization, 12, 197–205
  design, 196, 200–2
  non-therapeutic experimentation, 186–7, 190–1
  objectivity, 196–8, 202–3, 216
  risk to subjects, 186, 191–2
  value of, 195, 200, 203–5
respirators, 157, 167, 168–9
retirement, 11, 45–6, 64
  abilities, 133–4
  effects, 134–5
  history of, 131–4
  mandatory, 129–34
  post-retirement, 34
risk-taking, 208–13
Rowell-Sirois Commission, 144

SAAC. *See* Society for Applied Anthropology in Canada
Saikewicz case (Superior Court of Massachusetts), 172, 180
science: adaptation, 67–9; ethics, 69
self-esteem, 210
senility. *See* incompetence
sex differences, 62–3
Social Security Act, 135
social services, 18, 127, 129, 137–8
  Canada Assistance Plan, 144
society
  attitudes, 78
  common good, 187–90, 213
  rights, 127–8, 136–40
  values, 64
Society for Applied Anthropology in Canada (SAAC), 197, 201–5
socioeconomic status, 148, 194–5
  cognitive abilities, 57
Stoffman v. *Vancouver General Hospital*, 130
stress, 79–80
suffering, 38, 161–3, 174, 192

terminal decline, 57. *See also* euthanasia
time
  cognitive abilities, 58
  entropy, 66–7
  negentropy, 66–7

triage, 48–50

United States
- demographics, 98–9
- euthanasia, 159–63, 172–3, 175–82
- retirement, 129–32

United States Senate Committee on Human Resources, 131

verbal ability, 57

voluntarism, 48

Wechsler Adult Intelligence Scale, 57
welfare state, 128
wisdom, 60–1, 217–19
women
- health care, 148
- life expectancy, 63
- poverty, 44
- psychological health, 62–3

World Health Organization, 150–1

Index of Names

Achenbaum, W.A., 132
Acton, J.P., 35
Anderson, B.G., 80
Anderson, R., 68
Annas, G., 170n
Aquinas, T., 53n
Arenberg, D., 62
Atcheson, E., 141n
Atchley, R.C., 53n
Auger, J.A., 195, 196, 197, 200, 202, 203, 205
Avorn, J., 35, 78

Baltes, M.M., 80
Baltes, P.B., 73
Barnes, G.E., 146
Baron, C., 182n
Bayer, R., 96n
Bayley, C., 194, 196, 204
Beauchamp, T.L., 184, 195
Beiser, M., 65
Bengtson, V.L., 62, 78
Bennett, J.C., 41, 53n
Bennett, J.E., 145, 148
Bennett, K., 87
Bentham, J., 128
Berg, S., 62
Berkman, L.F., 148
Bird, R.M., 145
Birren, J.E., 57, 58, 59, 60, 61, 62, 65, 66, 68, 74, 216
Blandford, A.H., 146, 151n
Bleicher, J., 220
Bojanowski, B.C., 91, 96n
Bombardier, C., 96n
Bortner, R.W., 74
Botwinick, J., 56, 58, 59
Brandstadter, J., 76
Britton, J.H., 62
Britton, J.O., 62
Brody, E.M., 151
Brody, J., 40n
Bronte, L., 65, 67
Brown, E.R., 143
Browne, A., 182n
Bryden, K., 142, 143, 144
Butler, R.N., 32, 52n
Butt, S.D., 65

California Civil Code, 53n
Callahan, D., 53n, 96n, 170n
Casey, E., 218
Cassell, J., 198–200, 201
Cassidy, H.M., 142, 144
Cavanaugh, J.C., 59
Chandler, M.J., 75
Chappell, N.L., 143, 146, 151, 151n
Charness, N., 60
Childress, J.F., 184
Clark, M., 80
Clayton, V.P., 61
Cloyes, S.A., 26, 29
Coburn, D., 143, 146
Cohen, D., 146
Cohler, B., 217
Cole, T.R., 10

Collins, K., 145
Comfort, A., 55, 56
Commission on Compulsory Retirement (Manitoba), 129, 134n, 140n
Costa, P.T., 61, 62
Craik, F.I.M., 73
Crichton, A., 150
Cunningham, W.R., 66

Daniels, N., 96n
D'Arcy, D., 143
De Friese, G.H., 151
Deloria, V., 204
Denney, N.W., 73
Denton, F.T., 113, 115, 119, 122n
Dershowitz, A., 214n
Detsky, A.S., 145
Dittman-Kohli, F., 73
Dixon, R.A., 73
Dowd, J.J., 196, 205
Drummond, M., 89, 90, 91
Dubos, R.J., 94, 148

Edmund, L., 213
Ehrenreich, B., 148
Ehrenreich, J., 148
Eisendorfer, C., 146
Englehardt, H.T., 96n
Enos, D.D., 143, 144
Erikson, E.H., 61
Estes, C.L., 147, 148
Evans, R.G., 145, 151

Feaver, C.H., 122n
Feeny, D., 87
Feinberg, J., 96n
Fingerote, E., 213n
Finnis, J., 87
Firman, J.P., 156
Fletcher, J., 53n
Fraser, R.D., 145
Freeman, J.M., 38, 39
Fried, C., 96n
Friedson, E., 149
Fries, J.F., 33, 34

Garder, F.F., 57
Gee, E.U., 91, 96n
George, L.K., 62
Gillum, B., 62
Gillum, R., 62
Gouze, M., 62
Government of Canada, 145, 147
Graebner, W., 131, 132, 135
Grant, K.R., 148
Grubb, A., 86, 87
Gruman, G.J., 64, 65
Gutman, G.M., 91, 96n
Guttman, D., 146
Guyatt, G., 87

Hall, E., 84
Handler, P., 55, 56
Harris, R., 80
Hart, H.L.A., 128, 170n
Havighurst, R.J., 80
Hedlund, B., 68
Henig, R.M., 216
Hollister, R., 139
Honore, A.M., 170n
Huizer, G., 195, 197, 203
Hultsch, D.F., 74
Hunter, K.I., 80

Illich, I., 149
Irving, A., 143

Jacobs, A., 74, 75
Jarvie, I.C., 203, 206n
Jonas, H., 191

Kasschau, P.L., 62
Kastenbaum, R., 74, 216
Kaufert, J.M., 146
Kelman, H.C., 194, 195, 198, 200, 201, 204, 205, 206n
Kleiber, N., 198, 201, 201, 202, 203, 206n
Kohlberg, L., 81
Klockars, C.B., 201
Kluge, E.W., 88, 89, 94, 95
Krasny, J., 145, 148
Kuhn, M., 196
Kuypers, J.A., 78

Lachman, J.L., 59, 60
Lachman, R., 59, 60
Lalonde, M., 84
Landefeld, J.S., 35
Langer, E.J., 78
Lansing, A.I., 56
Law Reform Commission of Canada, 27, 156, 159, 160, 161, 162, 163, 168, 172, 173, 174, 175, 176, 177, 178,

181, 182
LeClair, M., 145
Lee, S.S., 145
Leman, C., 143
Leon, G.R., 62
Levin, J., 215
Levin, W., 215
Lewin, K., 202
Light, L., 198, 201, 201, 202, 203, 206n
Linn, M.W., 80
Livson, F., 62
Lonergan, B.J., 38
Lopate, C., 206n
Lowe, C.R., 148

McCormick, R., 186, 188, 189–90
McCrae, R.R., 61, 62
McGeer, A., 96n
MacIntyre, A., 181
McKeown, T., 148
McKinlay, J.B., 148
McKinlay, S.M., 148
MacLean, M.J., 139
Maguire, D., 52
Manga, P., 148
Maritain, J., 190
Marsh, L., 144
Marshall, V.W., 201
Maxwell, R., 148
May, W., 5, 13n, 51, 190
Mead, M., 197, 201
Metzger, R., 59
Miller, K., 59
Minister of Supply and Services 136
Mischel, W., 61
Mishler, E.G. 147, 149
Mitchell-Pederson, L., 213
Monge, R.H., 57
Morris, H., 209n
Moskop, J.C., 87
Mottet, D., 91, 96n
Mullins, L.C., 80

National Advisory Council on Aging, 29
National Commission for the Protection of Human Subjects, 192
National Council on Welfare, 136, 138
National Institute of Child Health and Human Development, 74
Neugarten, B.L., 61, 80, 149, 217
New, P., 143
Nezworski, T., 59
Nilsson, L.V., 62, 63
Nozik, R., 128

Obusek, C.J., 58
Odell, C.E., 131
Okum, M.A., 62

Parham, I.A., 62
Parliamentary Committee on Equality Rights, 129
Parliamentary Task Force on Pension Reform, 136, 138
Parsons, T., 198
Perlmutter, M., 58, 59
Persson, G., 63
Peterson, D.M., 146
Peterson, P.G., 62
Pickett, G., 78
Pifer, A., 65, 67
Polgar, S., 197
Poon, L.W., 73
Powell, C., 213
Prado, C.G., 218, 219, 221
Pratt, T.C., 80
President's Commission for the Study of Ethical Problems in Medicine and Biomedical and Behavioral Research, 86, 87, 96n, 156, 159, 160, 161, 162, 163, 164, 168, 172, 175, 176, 177, 178, 179, 180, 181, 182, 182n
Preston, R.P., 25

Rabbitt, P., 58
Rachels, J., 170n
Ragan, P.K., 62
Ramsey, P., 51, 91, 186, 190
Rappaport, J., 75
Ratzan, R., 183
Rawls, J., 128
Record, R.G., 148
Reich, W., 184, 190
Reiman, J.H., 198
Reisenzein, R., 80
Reichard, S., 62
Richardson, M., 197
Richmond, J., 30n
Rodin, J., 78
Rosenwaike, I., 40n
Rossie, I., 196
Royal Commission on Health Services in Canada, 84
Ryan, W., 195

Ryden, M.B., 80

Salthouse, T.A., 57
Schaie, K.W., 57, 62, 65, 73, 74, 216
Schneider, E., 40n
Schoepf, B.G., 195
Schwartz, R., 86, 87
Selye, H., 79
Seskin, E., 35n
Seigler, I.C., 62
Sinclair, A.J., 96n
Smith, D.H., 53n
Society for Applied Anthropology in Canada, 197, 201, 202, 203, 205
Soelle, D., 26, 29
Spencer, B.G., 113, 115, 119, 122n
Stafford, J.L., 60
Statistics Canada, 85, 86, 147
Steinbock, B., 170n
Stone, L.O., 139
Storandt, M., 59
Strain, L.A., 146, 151n
Strickland, B.R., 80
Strother, C.R., 62
Sullivan, L., 141n
Sultan, P., 143, 144
Suzman, R., 40n
Syme, S.L., 148

Thomae, H., 62
Tindale, J.A., 201
Tobin, S.S., 80
Torrance, G.W., 96n, 143, 146
Tsalikis, G., 146
Tugwell, P., 87
Tulkin, S.R., 74
Turner, R.D., 148
Tyler, L.E., 67

U.S. Department of Labor, 141n

Vladeck, B.C., 150

Wagar, W.W., 69
Warren, R.M., 58
Wax, M.C., 205n
Welford, A.T., 58
Weller, G.R., 148
White-Riley, M., 40n
Whittaker, E., 202, 203, 205n
Willems, E.P., 80, 81
Williams, G., 217
Williams, M.V., 57,60
Willis, S.L., 73, 74
Wilson, L., 143
Winkler, E., 170n
Winslow, G.R., 49, 50
Wolfson, A.D., 96n
Woodruff, D.S., 62, 74
Woods, A.M., 57, 60
Woomert, A., 151